The ultimate Dash Diet Cookbook for Beginners

A Comprehensive Guide to Lowering Blood Pressure, Slowing Aging, and Boosting Your Immune System

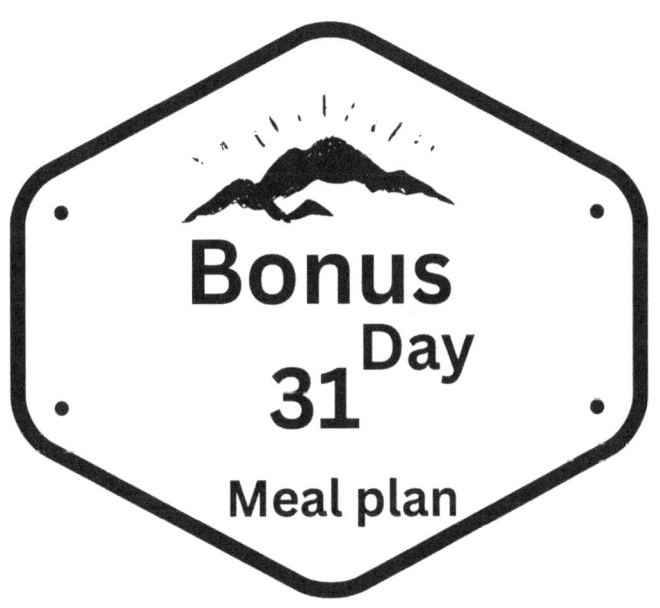

Bonus
31 **Day**
Meal plan

By

Melissa B. Kimbrell

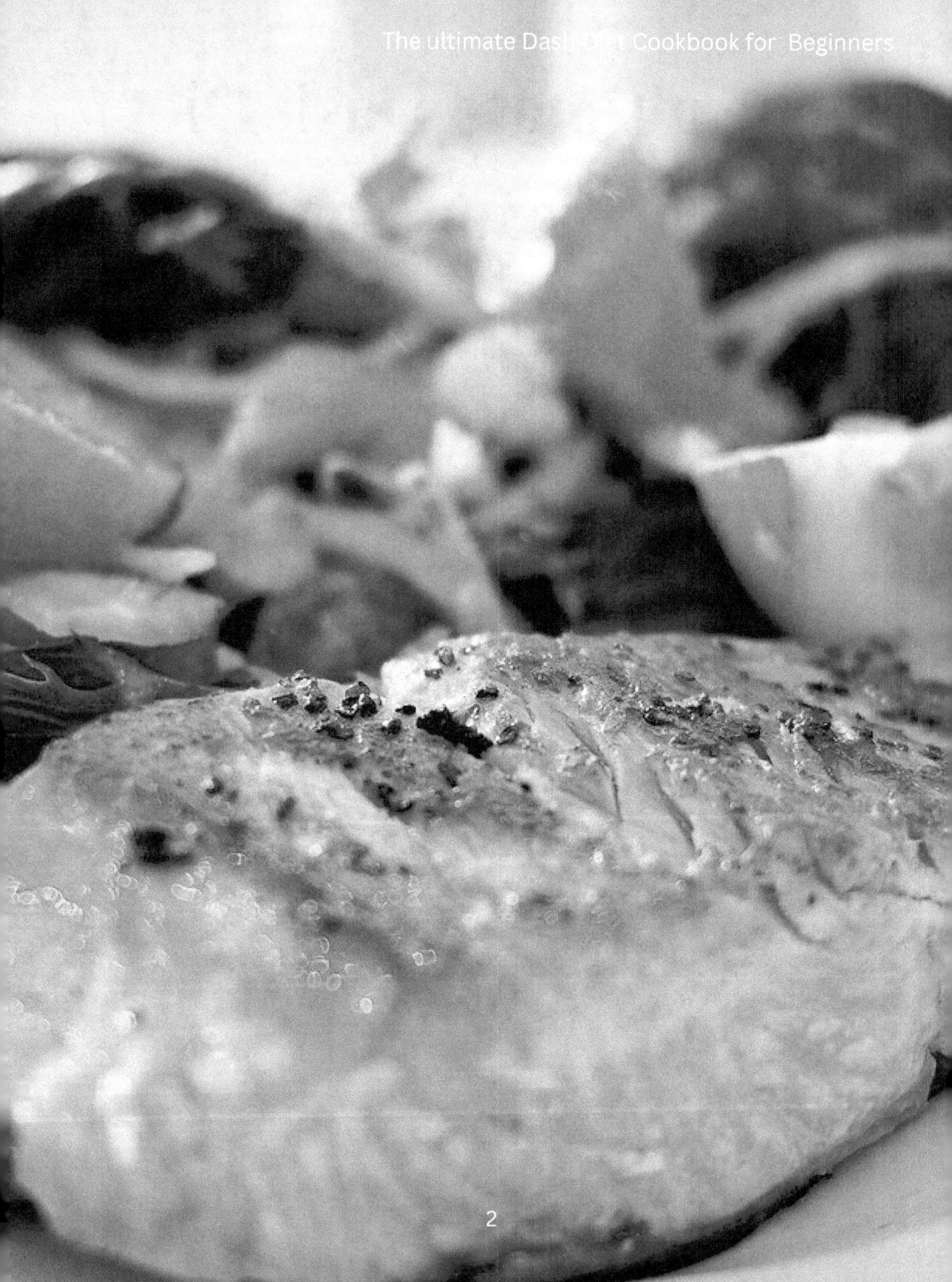

Copyright© 2023 by Melissa B. Kimbrell

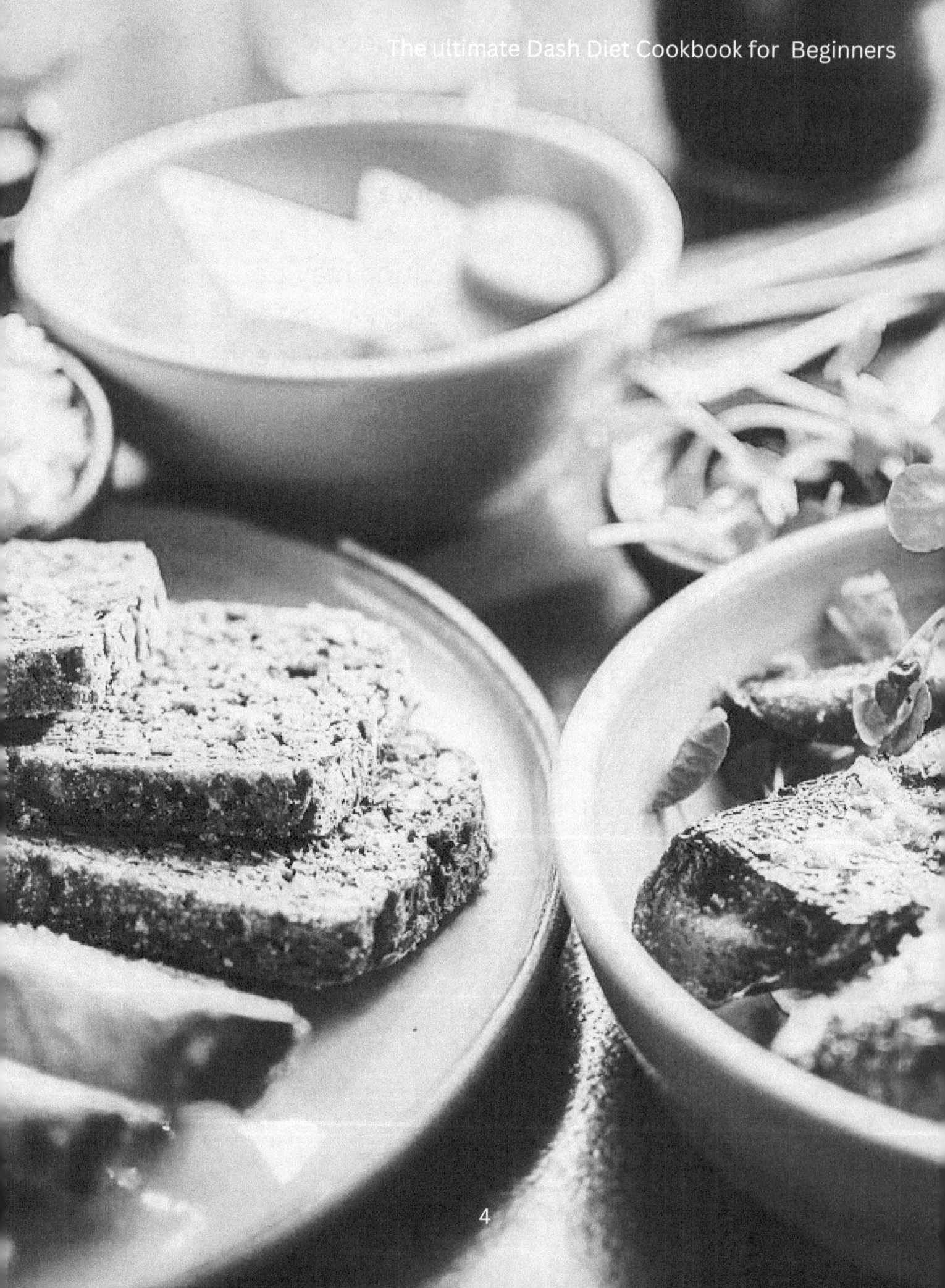

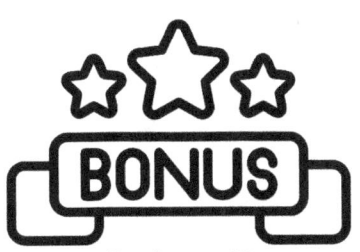

Here is your 31- day meal plan
All recipes are covered in the book

Day 1

Breakfast
Overnight oats with berries and nuts

Lunch
Salad with grilled chicken or fish

Dinner
Baked salmon with roasted vegetables

Day 2

Breakfast
Whole-wheat toast with avocado and eggs

Lunch
Lentil soup

Dinner
Turkey and vegetable stir-fry

Day 3

Breakfast
Greek yogurt with fruit and granola

Lunch
Tuna salad sandwich on whole-wheat bread

Dinner
Chicken chili

Day 4

Breakfast
Smoothie with fruit, yogurt, and protein powder

Lunch
Salad with grilled tofu or tempeh

Dinner
Black bean soup with cornbread

Day 5

Breakfast
Whole-wheat pancakes with fruit and syrup

Lunch
Veggie burger on a whole-wheat bun

Dinner
Baked cod with roasted vegetables

Day 6

Breakfast
Scrambled eggs with spinach and cheese

Lunch
Chicken salad sandwich on whole-wheat bread

Dinner
Salmon with lemon and dill

Day 7

Breakfast

Fruit and yogurt parfait

Lunch

Salad with grilled chicken or fish

Dinner

Vegetarian chili with cornbread

Day 8

Breakfast

Whole-wheat toast with avocado and eggs

Lunch

Lentil soup

Dinner

Turkey burgers with roasted sweet potatoes

Day 9

Breakfast

Greek yogurt with fruit and granola

Lunch

Tuna salad sandwich on whole-wheat bread

Dinner

Chicken stir-fry with brown rice

Day 10

Breakfast

Smoothie with fruit, yogurt, and protein powder

Lunch

Salad with grilled tofu or tempeh

Dinner

Black bean soup with cornbread

Day 11

Breakfast

Whole-wheat pancakes with fruit and syrup

Lunch

Veggie burger on a whole-wheat bun

Dinner

Baked cod with roasted vegetables

Day 12

Breakfast

Scrambled eggs with spinach and cheese

Lunch

Chicken salad sandwich on whole-wheat bread

Dinner

Salmon with lemon and dill

Day 13

Breakfast

Fruit and yogurt parfait

Lunch

Salad with grilled chicken or fish

Dinner

Vegetarian chili with cornbread

Day 14

Breakfast

Whole-wheat toast with avocado and eggs

Lunch

Lentil soup

Dinner

Turkey burgers with roasted sweet potatoes

Day 15

Breakfast

Greek yogurt with fruit and granola

Lunch

Tuna salad sandwich on whole-wheat bread

Dinner

Chicken stir-fry with brown rice

Day 16

Breakfast
Smoothie with fruit, yogurt, and protein powder

Lunch
Salad with grilled tofu or tempeh

Dinner
Black bean soup with cornbread

Day 17

Breakfast
Whole-wheat pancakes with fruit and syrup

Lunch
Veggie burger on a whole-wheat bun

Dinner
Baked cod with roasted vegetables

Day 18

Breakfast
Scrambled eggs with spinach and cheese

Lunch
Chicken salad sandwich on whole-wheat bread

Dinner
Salmon with lemon and dill

Day 19

Breakfast
Fruit and yogurt parfait

Lunch
Salad with grilled chicken or fish

Dinner
Vegetarian chili with cornbread

Day 20

Breakfast
Whole-wheat toast with avocado and eggs

Lunch
Lentil soup

Dinner
Turkey and vegetable stir-fry

Day 21

Breakfast
Greek yogurt with fruit and granola

Lunch
Tuna salad sandwich on whole-wheat bread

Dinner
Chicken chili

Day 22

Breakfast
Smoothie with fruit, yogurt, and protein powder

Lunch
Salad with grilled tofu or tempeh

Dinner
Black bean soup with cornbread

Day 23

Breakfast
Whole-wheat pancakes with fruit and syrup

Lunch
Veggie burger on a whole-wheat bun

Dinner
Baked cod with roasted vegetables

Day 24

Breakfast
Scrambled eggs with spinach and cheese

Lunch
Chicken salad sandwich on whole-wheat bread

Dinner
Salmon with lemon and dill

Day 25

Breakfast

Fruit and yogurt parfait

Lunch

Salad with grilled chicken or fish

Dinner

Vegetarian chili with cornbread

Day 26

Breakfast

Whole-wheat toast with avocado and eggs

Lunch

Lentil soup

Dinner

Turkey burgers with roasted sweet potatoes

Day 27

Breakfast

Greek yogurt with fruit and granola

Lunch

Tuna salad sandwich on whole-wheat bread

Dinner

Chicken stir-fry with brown rice

Day 28

Breakfast

Smoothie with fruit, yogurt, and protein powder

Lunch

Salad with grilled tofu or tempeh

Dinner

Black bean soup with cornbread

Day 29

Breakfast

Whole-wheat pancakes with fruit and syrup

Lunch

Veggie burger on a whole-wheat bun

Dinner

Baked cod with roasted vegetables

Day 30

Breakfast

Scrambled eggs with spinach and cheese

Lunch

Chicken salad sandwich on whole-wheat bread

Dinner

Salmon with lemon and dill

Day 31

Breakfast

Fruit and yogurt parfait

Lunch

Salad with grilled chicken or fish

Dinner

Vegetarian chili with cornbread

Table of contents

Let's dive into it

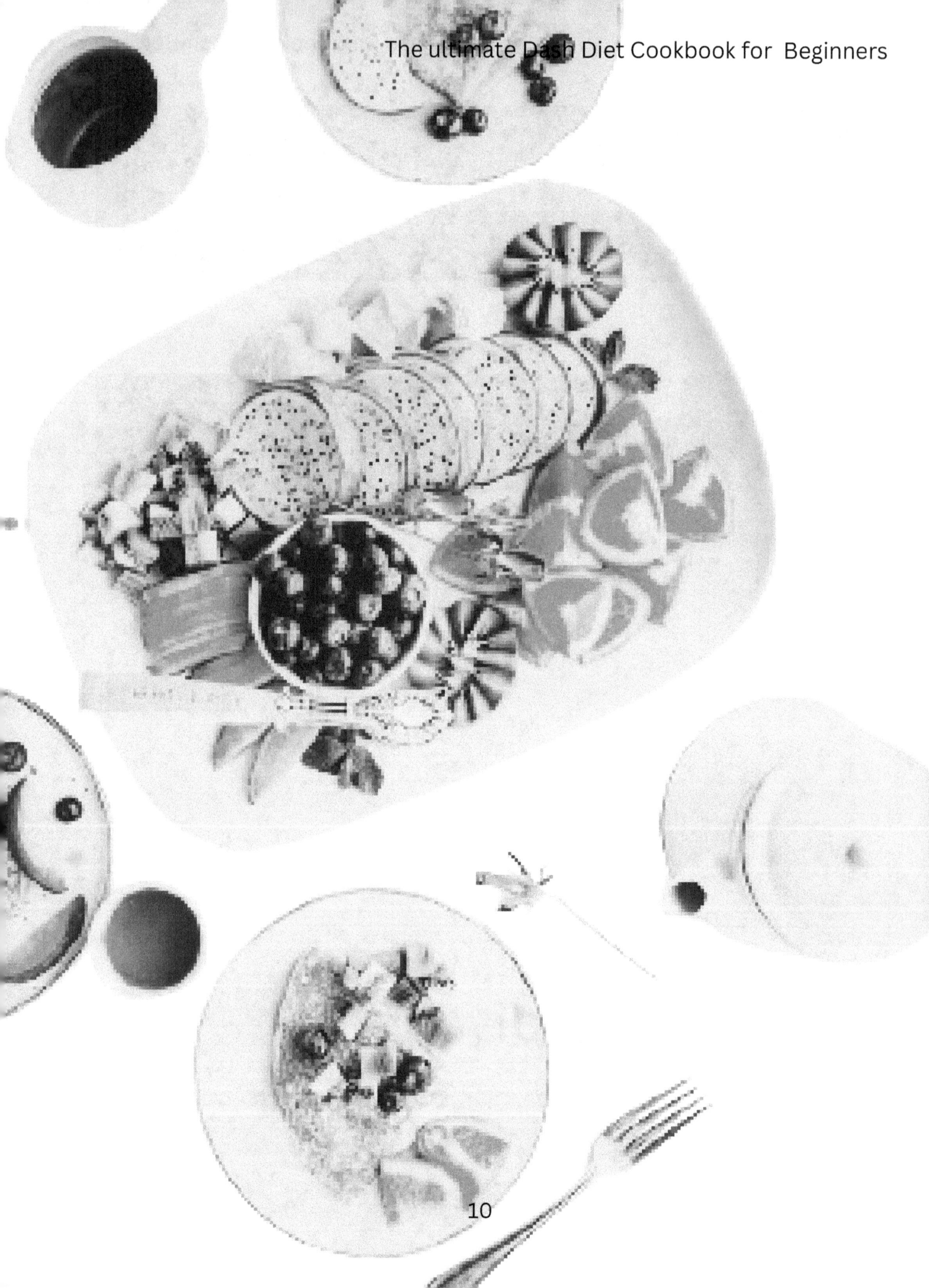

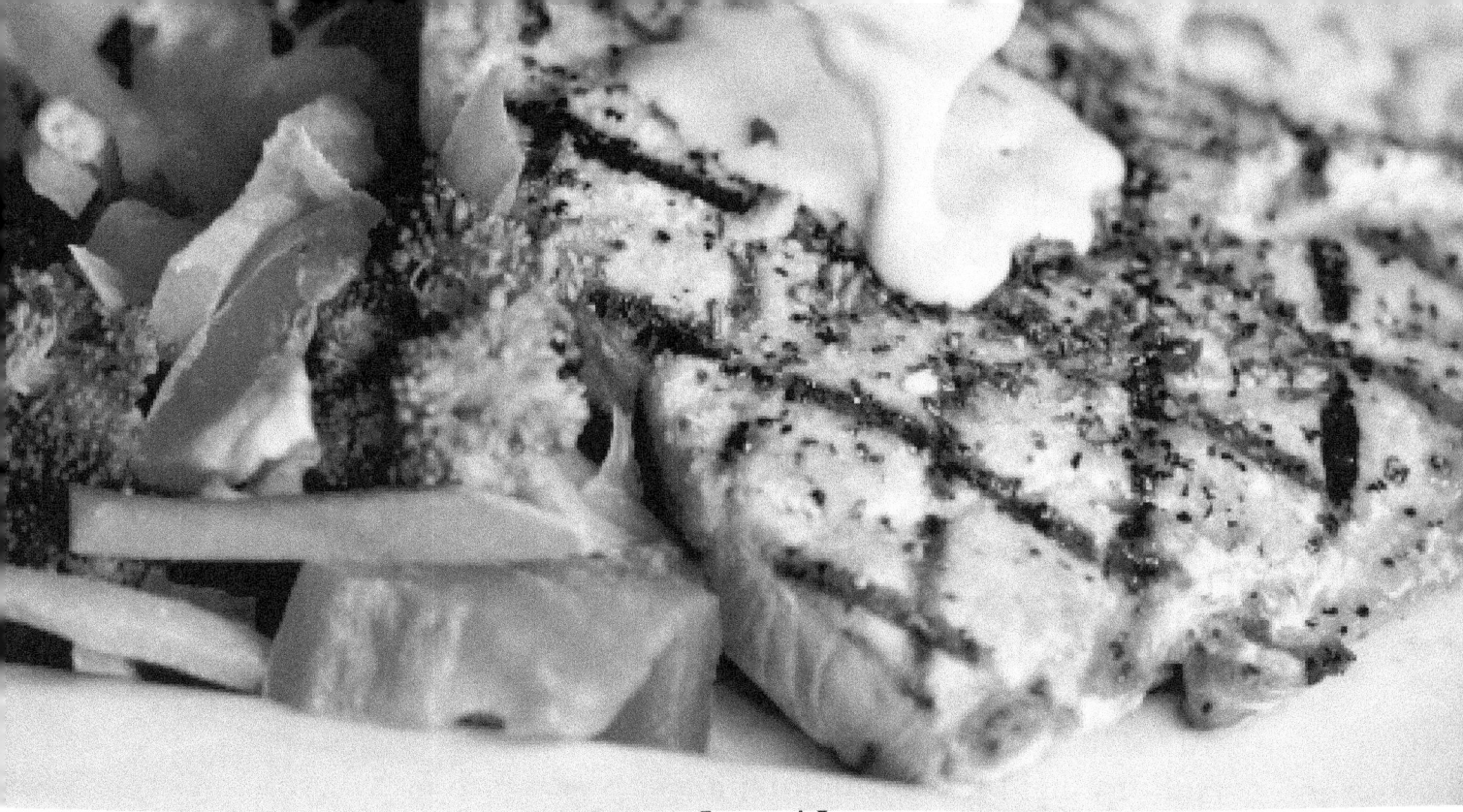

Introduction

In a world where chronic diseases like heart disease, stroke, and obesity are on the rise, it's more important than ever to take charge of your health. And one of the most effective ways to do that is by adopting a healthy diet. The DASH Diet Cookbook for Beginners is your comprehensive guide to lowering blood pressure, slowing aging, and boosting your immune system with the power of food.

What is the DASH Diet?

The DASH (Dietary Approaches to Stop Hypertension) dict is a scientifically proven eating plan that was developed by the National Institutes of Health (NIH) to lower blood pressure.

It has been shown to be incredibly effective, reducing blood pressure by an average of 8-14 mmHg in people with hypertension and 5-7 mmHg in people with normal blood pressure.

How Does the DASH Diet Work?

The DASH diet works by reducing sodium intake and increasing consumption of fruits, vegetables, whole grains, and low-fat dairy products. These foods are rich in potassium, magnesium, calcium, and fiber, all of which play a role in regulating blood pressure.

By limiting sodium, which can raise blood pressure, and incorporating these nutrient-rich foods, the DASH diet helps to keep blood pressure in a healthy range.

Benefits Beyond Blood Pressure

While the primary focus of the DASH diet is to lower blood pressure, its benefits extend far beyond that. Research has shown that the DASH diet can also:

- Reduce the risk of heart disease
- Decrease the risk of stroke
- Improve kidney function
- Slow down the aging process
- Strengthen the immune system
- Aid in weight loss or maintenance

Who Should Follow the DASH Diet?

The DASH diet is suitable for people of all ages and health conditions. It's particularly beneficial for those with high blood pressure, heart disease, or a family history of these conditions. However, even healthy individuals can reap the benefits of the DASH diet by adopting its healthy and nutritious eating habits.

How to Use This Cookbook

This cookbook is designed to provide you with everything you need to know about the DASH diet and how to incorporate it into your lifestyle. It includes:

- A comprehensive overview of the DASH diet and its benefits
- Delicious and easy-to-follow recipes for every meal, including breakfast, lunch, dinner, and snacks
- Tips for grocery shopping and meal planning
- Strategies for maintaining a DASH diet lifestyle
- A 31-day meal plan to help you get started

With the help of this cookbook, you'll embark on a journey towards a healthier, happier, and more vibrant you. Embrace the DASH diet and discover the power of food to transform your health and well-being.

Understanding Blood Pressure and the DASH Diet

Chapter 1 :

The Silent Killer: Understanding Blood Pressure

Blood pressure is the force of your blood pushing against the walls of your arteries. It's measured in two numbers: systolic and diastolic. Systolic pressure is the pressure when your heart beats, while diastolic pressure is the pressure when your heart is at rest.

Why is blood pressure important?

Blood pressure is important because it helps deliver oxygen and nutrients to your organs. If your blood pressure is too high or too low, it can damage your organs and lead to serious health problems.

What are the normal ranges of blood pressure?

The normal range for blood pressure is less than 120/80 mmHg. If your blood pressure is consistently 140/90 mmHg or higher, you have high blood pressure (hypertension). High blood pressure is a major risk factor for heart disease, stroke, kidney disease, and other health problems.

What are the signs and symptoms of high blood pressure?

Most people with high blood pressure don't have any symptoms. This is why it's often called the "silent killer." The only way to know for sure if you have high blood pressure is to get your blood pressure checked regularly.

What can you do to lower your blood pressure?

There are a number of things you can do to lower your blood pressure, including:

- Eating a healthy diet
- Exercising regularly
- Maintaining a healthy weight
- Limiting sodium intake
- Managing stress
- Quitting smoking

Chapter 2

The Role of Sodium in Blood Pressure Regulation

Sodium is a mineral that is found in many foods. It's essential for the body to function properly, but too much sodium can raise blood pressure. The American Heart Association recommends that adults limit their sodium intake to less than 2,300 milligrams per day.

How does sodium raise blood pressure?

When you eat sodium, your body holds onto extra fluid. This extra fluid puts more pressure on your arteries, which raises your blood pressure.

What are some sources of sodium?

Sodium is found in a variety of foods, including:
- Processed foods
- Restaurant meals
- Salty snacks
- Cured meats
- Canned foods
- Bread and pastries

How can you reduce your sodium intake?

There are a number of things you can do to reduce your sodium intake, including:

- Read food labels carefully and choose foods that are low in sodium.
- Cook more meals at home and use less salt.
- Limit your intake of processed foods, restaurant meals, and salty snacks.
- Choose fresh or frozen vegetables instead of canned vegetables.
- Rinse canned vegetables before eating them.
- Use herbs and spices to flavor your food instead of salt
- Taste your food before adding salt.

Chapter 3

How the DASH Diet Helps to Lower Blood Pressure

The DASH diet is a scientifically proven eating plan that can help to lower blood pressure. It's rich in fruits, vegetables, whole grains, and low-fat dairy products. These foods are low in sodium and high in potassium, magnesium, calcium, and fiber, all of which play a role in regulating blood pressure.

The DASH diet helps to lower blood pressure in a number of ways, including:
- Reducing sodium intake
- Increasing potassium intake

- Increasing magnesium intake
- Increasing calcium intake
- Increasing fiber intake

How much sodium does the DASH diet recommend?

The DASH diet recommends that adults limit their sodium intake to less than 2,300 milligrams per day. For people with high blood pressure, the DASH diet recommends limiting sodium intake to less than 1,500 milligrams per day.

What are some DASH-approved foods?

Here are some examples of DASH-approved foods:
- Fruits: Apples, bananas, berries, citrus fruits, melons
- Vegetables: Broccoli, carrots, leafy greens, potatoes, tomatoes
- Whole grains: Brown rice, oats, quinoa, whole-wheat bread
- Low-fat dairy products: Fat-free milk, yogurt, cheese
- Lean protein: Fish, chicken, beans, lentils
- Nuts and seeds: Almonds, cashews, sunflower seeds

What are some DASH-discouraged foods?

DASH-discouraged foods includes:

- Processed foods
- Bacon
- chips
- cookies
- crackers

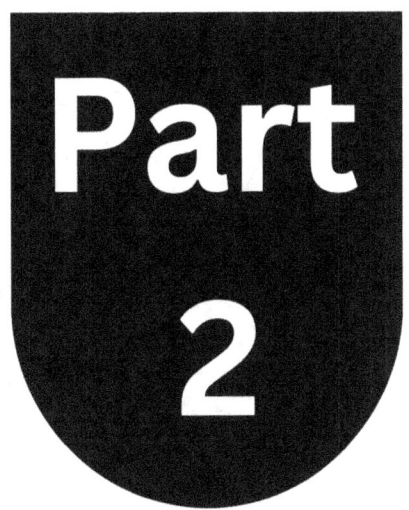

Part 2

Delicious DASH Diet Recipes for Every Meal

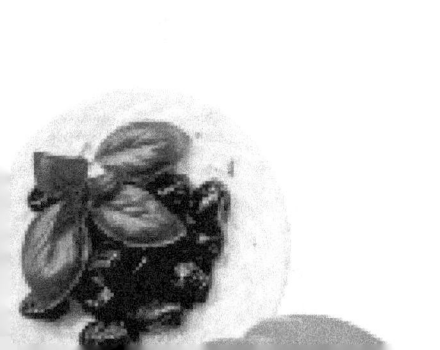
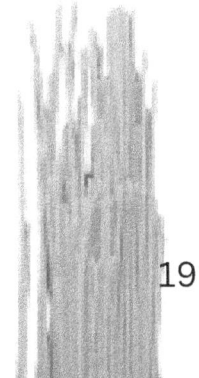
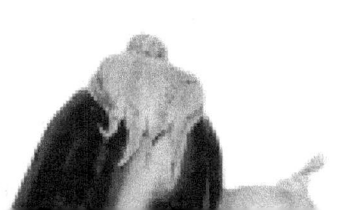

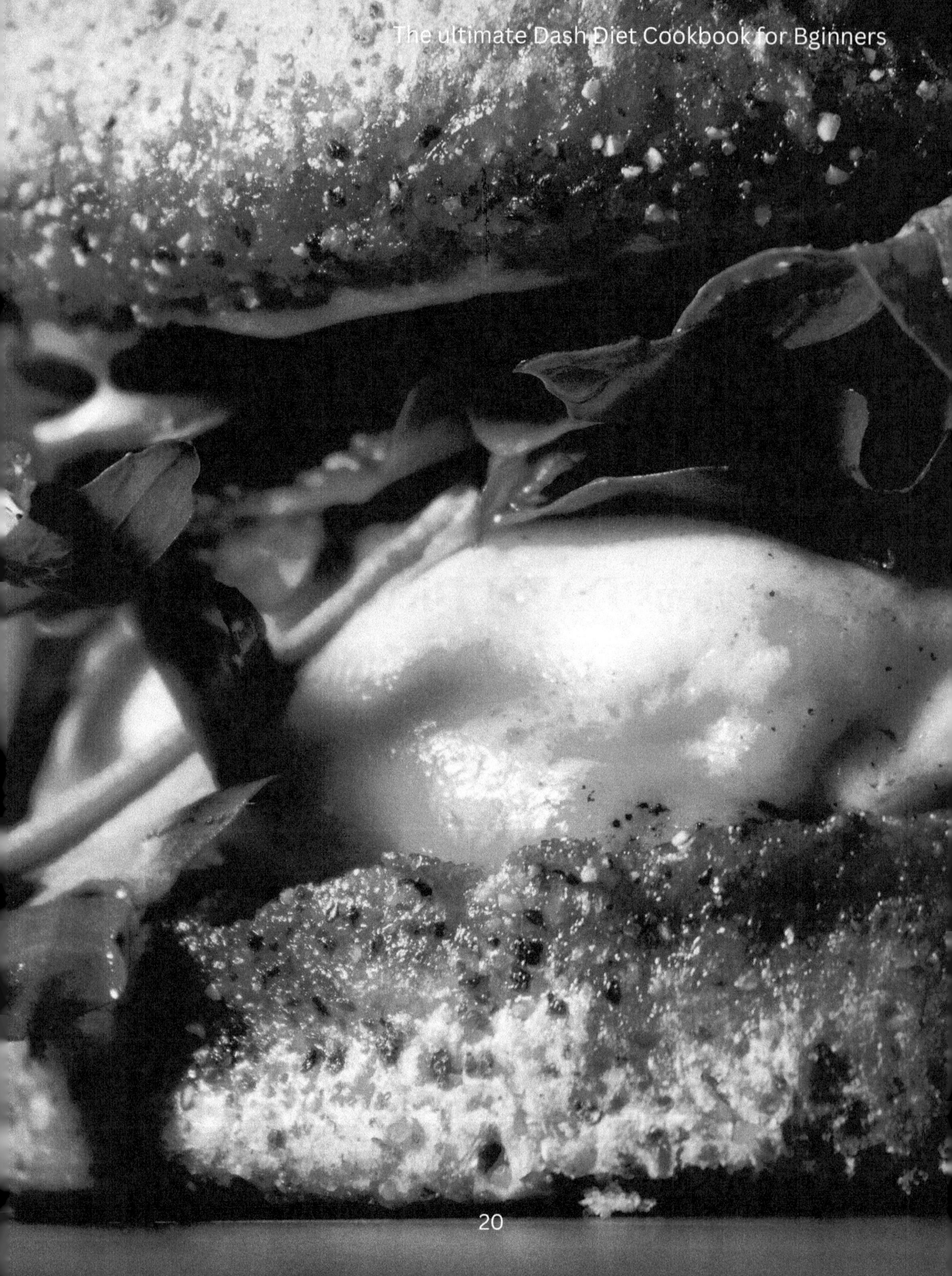

Breakfast

Start your day with a nourishing DASH-friendly breakfast

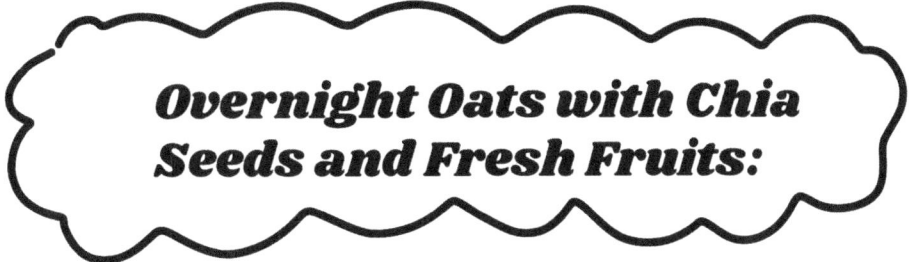

Overnight Oats with Chia Seeds and Fresh Fruits:

This easy-to-prepare recipe combines the fiber and protein from oats with the omega-3 fatty acids from chia seeds and the antioxidants from fresh fruits, making it a power-packed breakfast option.

Recipe

Preparation Time: 5 minutes	Cooking Time: None	Serving Size: 1 cup

Nutritional Information per Serving

Calories: 350 (without toppings) Protein: 16g Fiber: 8g Calcium: 5g

Ingredients;

- ½ cup rolled oats
- ¼ cup chia seeds
- 1 cup unsweetened soy milk or almond milk
- ½ cup mixed berries (strawberries, blueberries, raspberries)
- 1 tablespoon honey
- A pinch of cinnamon

Instructions:

1. In a jar or container, combine the oats, chia seeds, milk, and yogurt. Stir well until all ingredients are combined.
2. Cover the jar or container and refrigerate overnight.
3. In the morning, stir the oats and add your desired toppings. Serve immediately.

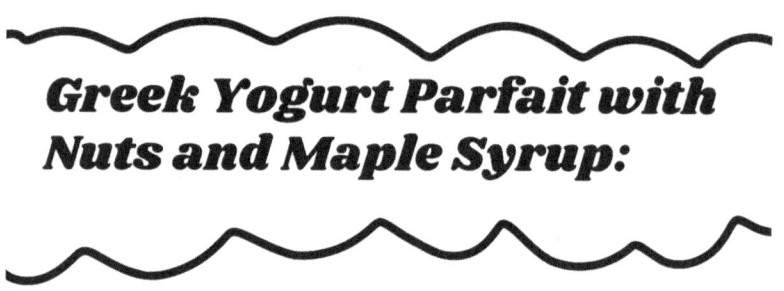

Greek Yogurt Parfait with Nuts and Maple Syrup:

This layered parfait is a delightful treat that combines the creamy texture of Greek yogurt with the crunch of nuts and the sweetness of maple syrup.

Recipe

Preparation Time: 5 minutes	Cooking Time: None	Serving Size: 1 cup

Nutritional Information per Serving

Calories: 300, Protein: 20g, Fat: 10g, Carbohydrates: 30g
Fiber: 5g, Sugar: 15g

Ingredients;

- 1 cup plain Greek yogurt
- 1/2 cup mixed nuts, chopped
- 2 tablespoons maple syrup
- 1/4 cup fresh fruit, sliced

Instructions:

1. In a glass or bowl, layer the Greek yogurt, nuts, maple syrup, and fresh fruit.
2. Stir gently to combine.
3. Enjoy immediately!

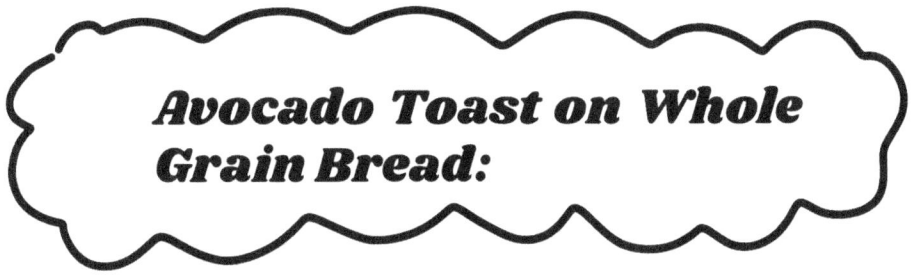

Avocado Toast on Whole Grain Bread:

This simple yet satisfying breakfast combines the healthy fats from avocado with the fiber from whole grain bread, providing a balanced and nutritious start to the day.

Recipe

Preparation Time: 5 minutes	Cooking Time: None	Serving Size: 1 slice

Nutritional Information per Serving

Calories: 250, Protein: 8g, Fat: 10g, Carbohydrates: 30g, Fiber: 8g, Sugar: 2g

Ingredients;

- 1 slice whole grain bread
- 1/2 ripe avocado, mashed
- 1 teaspoon lemon juice
- Salt and pepper to taste

Instructions:

1. Toast the bread to your desired level of doneness.
2. In a small bowl, mash the avocado with lemon juice, salt, and pepper.
3. Spread the avocado mixture evenly over the toasted bread.

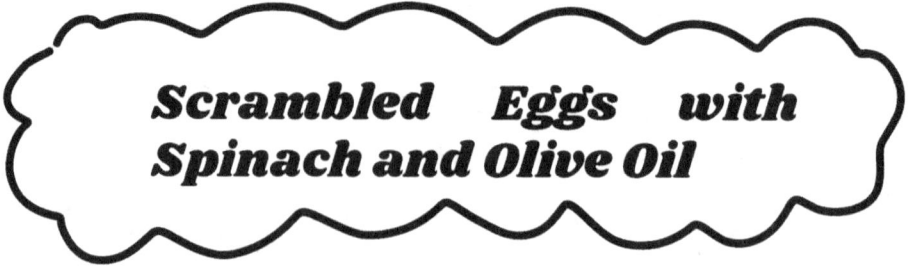

Scrambled Eggs with Spinach and Olive Oil

This protein-rich breakfast is packed with spinach's vitamins and minerals and enhanced by the healthy fats from olive oil.

Recipe

Preparation Time: 5 minutes	Cooking Time: 5 min	Serving Size: 1

Nutritional Information per Serving

Calories: 200, Protein: 15g, Fat: 10g, Carbohydrates: 2g, Fiber: 1g

Ingredients;

- 2 large eggs
- 1 tablespoon olive oil
- 1/2 cup baby spinach
- Salt and pepper to taste

Instructions:

1. In a medium bowl, whisk together the eggs.
2. Heat the olive oil in a small skillet over medium heat.
3. Add the spinach to the skillet and cook until wilted, about 2 minutes.
4. Add the eggs to the skillet and cook, stirring constantly, until the eggs are set to your desired doneness.
5. Season with salt and pepper to taste.
6. Serve immediately.

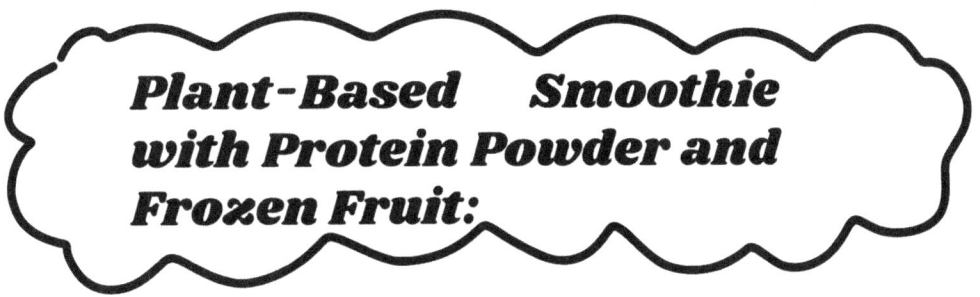

Plant-Based Smoothie with Protein Powder and Frozen Fruit:

This refreshing and energizing smoothie provides a blend of plant-based protein, fiber, and vitamins, making it an ideal breakfast option for those on the go.

Recipe

Preparation Time: 5 minutes	Cooking Time: None	Serving Size: 1

Nutritional Information per Serving

Calories: 300, Protein: 20g, Fat: 5g   Carbohydrates: 40g, Fiber: 5g, Sugar: 15g

Ingredients;

- cup unsweetened plant-based milk
- 1 banana, frozen
- 1 cup frozen mixed berries
- 1 scoop plant-based protein powder

Instructions:

1. In a blender, combine the plant-based milk, frozen banana, frozen mixed berries, and protein powder.
2. Blend until smooth and creamy.
3. Serve immediately.

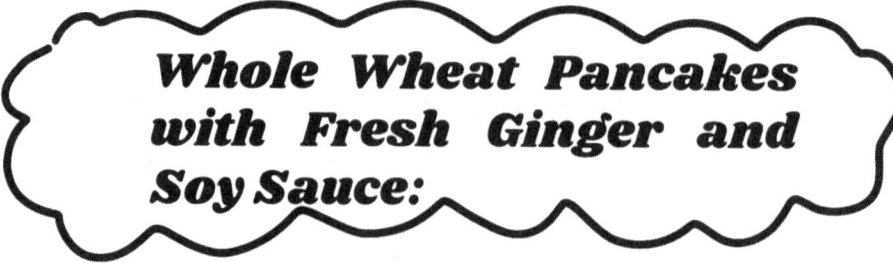

Whole Wheat Pancakes with Fresh Ginger and Soy Sauce:

These pancakes are a savory twist on a classic breakfast dish, offering a unique flavor profile and a boost of fiber from whole wheat flour.

Recipe

Preparation Time: 10 minutes	Cooking Time: 10 minutes	Serving Size: 4 pancakes

Nutritional Information per Serving

Calories: 250, Protein: 5g, Fat: 10g.   Carbohydrates: 35g, Fiber: 5g, Sugar: 10g

Ingredients;

- 1 cup whole wheat flour
- 1 teaspoon baking powder
- 1/2 teaspoon baking soda
- 1/4 teaspoon salt
- 1 tablespoon sugar
- 1 tablespoon ground ginger
- 1/2 cup soy sauce
- 1 cup water
- 1 tablespoon vegetable oil

Instructions:

1. In a large bowl, whisk together the dry ingredients: flour, baking powder, baking soda, salt, sugar, and ginger.
2. In a separate bowl, whisk together the wet ingredients: soy sauce, water, and vegetable oil.
3. Pour the wet ingredients into the dry ingredients and whisk until just combined.
4. Heat a griddle or large skillet over medium heat. Grease the pan with cooking spray or butter.

5. Pour 1/4 cup of batter onto the griddle for each pancake.

6. Cook for 2-3 minutes per side, or until golden brown.

7. Serve immediately with your favorite toppings, such as fresh fruit, maple syrup, or whipped cream.

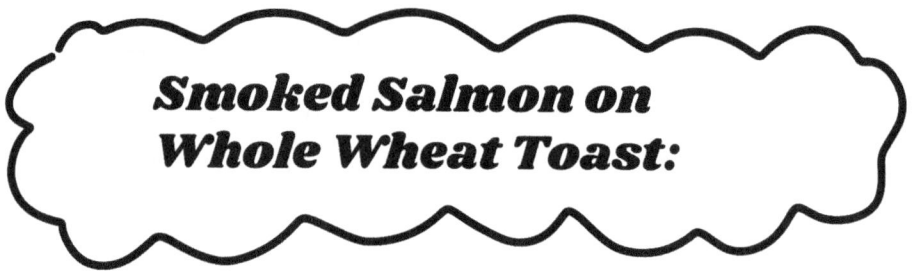

Smoked Salmon on Whole Wheat Toast:

This elegant and flavorful breakfast is rich in protein and omega-3 fatty acids from smoked salmon, complemented by the fiber from whole wheat toast.

Recipe

Preparation Time: 5 minutes	Cooking Time: None	Serving Size: 1

Nutritional Information per Serving

Calories: 300, Protein: 15g, Fat: 10g. Carbohydrates: 30g, Fiber: 5g, Sodium: 500mg

Ingredients;

- 2 slices whole wheat bread
- 4 ounces smoked salmon, thinly sliced
- 1 tablespoon cream cheese, softened
- 1 tablespoon lemon juice
- Salt and pepper to taste

Instructions:

1. Toast the bread to your desired level of doneness.
2. In a small bowl, mix together the cream cheese, lemon juice, salt, and pepper.
3. Spread the cream cheese mixture evenly over the toasted bread.
4. Top with smoked salmon slices.

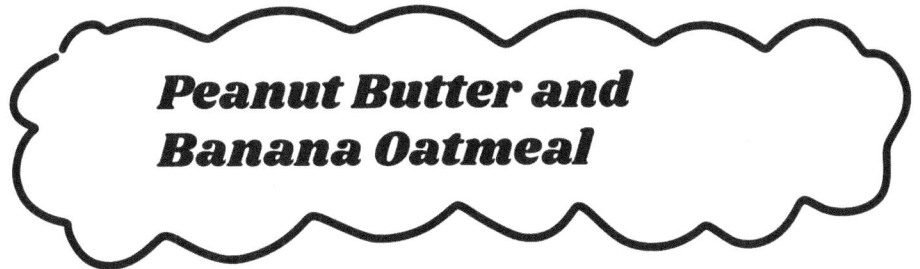

Peanut Butter and Banana Oatmeal

This classic breakfast combination provides a satisfying balance of protein, fiber, and healthy fats, keeping you energized throughout the morning.

Recipe

Preparation Time: 5 minutes	Cooking Time: 5 minutes	Serving Size: 1

Nutritional Information per Serving

Calories: 350, Protein: 10g, Fat: 15g, Carbohydrates: 45g, Fiber: 5g, Sugar: 10g

Ingredients;

- 1/2 cup rolled oats
- 1 cup water or milk
- 1/4 cup peanut butter
- 1/2 banana, mashed
- 1 teaspoon cinnamon
- Honey or maple syrup (optional)

Instructions:

1. In a small saucepan, combine oats, water or milk, and peanut butter.
2. Bring to a boil over medium heat, then reduce heat and simmer for 5 minutes, or until oats are cooked through.
3. Stir in mashed banana and cinnamon.
4. Sweeten with honey or maple syrup to taste, if desired.

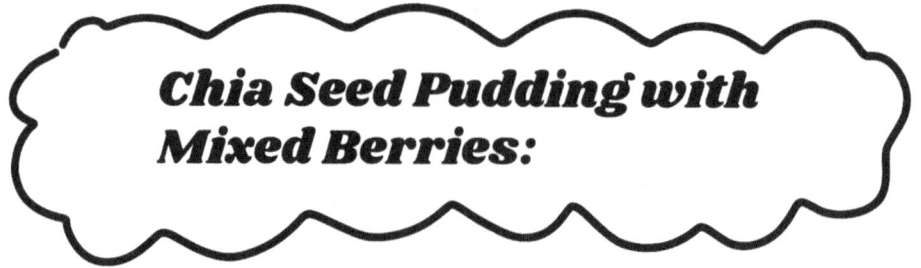

Chia Seed Pudding with Mixed Berries:

This pudding is a nutrient-dense and versatile breakfast option, offering a rich source of fiber, protein, and omega-3 fatty acids from chia seeds, along with the antioxidants from mixed berries.

Recipe

Preparation Time: 5 minutes	Cooking Time: None	Serving Size: 1

Nutritional Information per Serving

Calories: 250, Protein: 6g, Fat: 15g
Carbohydrates: 20g, Fiber: 10g, Sugar: 5g

Ingredients;

- 1/2 cup chia seeds
- 1 cup milk of your choice
- 1/4 cup mixed berries, frozen or fresh
- 1 tablespoon maple syrup or honey (optional)
- 1 teaspoon vanilla extract

Instructions:

1. In a small bowl or jar, combine the chia seeds, milk, mixed berries, maple syrup or honey (if using), and vanilla extract.
2. Stir until well combined.
3. Cover and refrigerate for at least 30 minutes, or overnight.
4. When ready to serve, stir the chia seed pudding again and top with additional mixed berries, if desired.

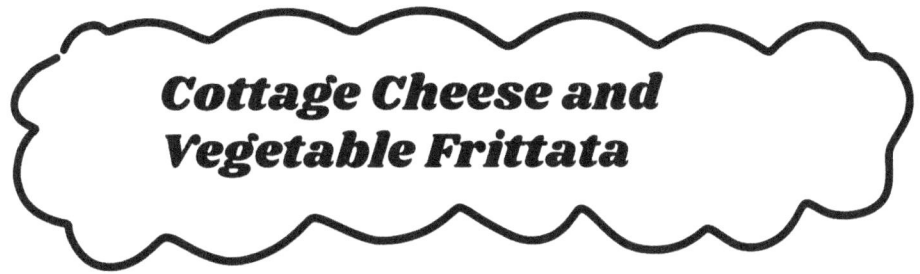

Cottage Cheese and Vegetable Frittata

This frittata is a protein-packed and fiber-rich breakfast that combines the savory flavors of cottage cheese with the nutrient-dense goodness of vegetables.

Recipe

Preparation Time: 10 minutes	Cooking Time: 20 minutes	Serving Size: 4

Nutritional Information per Serving

Calories: 300, Protein: 18g, Fat: 15g
Carbohydrates: 10g, Fiber: 2g, Sodium: 400mg

Ingredients;

- 1 tablespoon olive oil
- 1/2 cup chopped onion
- 1 cup chopped vegetables of your choice (such as bell peppers, mushrooms, spinach)
- 2 cloves garlic, minced
- 4 large eggs
- 3/4 cup cottage cheese
- 1/2 cup grated Parmesan cheese
- Kosher salt and freshly ground black pepper to taste

Instructions:

1. Preheat the oven to 375°F (190°C).
2. Heat olive oil in a large oven-safe skillet over medium heat. Add onion and cook until softened, about 5 minutes.
3. Add chopped vegetables and cook until tender, about 5 minutes more.
4. Add garlic and cook for 30 seconds more, until fragrant.
5. In a large bowl, whisk together eggs, cottage cheese, Parmesan cheese, salt, and pepper.

6. Pour egg mixture into the skillet with the vegetables.

7. Transfer the skillet to the oven and bake for 20 minutes, or until the eggs are set and the top is golden brown.

8. Let the frittata cool for a few minutes before cutting into wedges and serving.

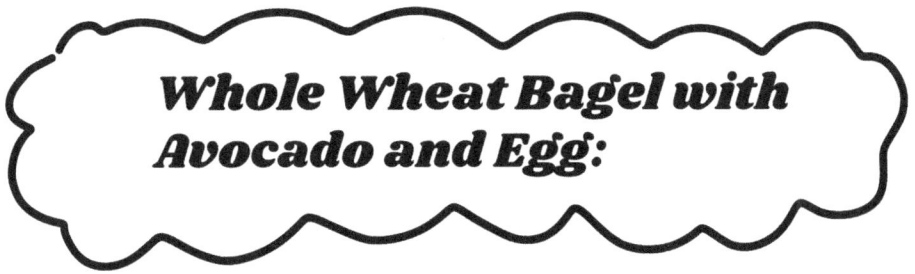

Whole Wheat Bagel with Avocado and Egg:

This bagel sandwich is a hearty and satisfying breakfast option, combining the fiber from whole wheat bread with the healthy fats from avocado and the protein from an egg.

Recipe

Preparation Time: 5 minutes	Cooking Time: 5 minutes	Serving Size: 1

Nutritional Information per Serving

Calories: 350, Protein: 15g, Fat: 15g   Carbohydrates: 40g, Fiber: 8g, Sugar: 3g

Ingredients;

- 1 whole-wheat bagel, toasted
- 1/2 ripe avocado, mashed
- 1 tablespoon lemon juice
- Salt and pepper to taste
- 1 large egg
- 1 teaspoon olive oil
- Optional toppings: sliced tomatoes, red onion, hot sauce

Instructions:

1. Toast the bagel until lightly golden brown.
2. In a small bowl, mash the avocado with lemon juice, salt, and pepper.
3. Spread the avocado mixture evenly over the toasted bagel.
4. Heat the olive oil in a small skillet over medium heat.
5. Crack the egg into the skillet and cook to your desired doneness.
6. Place the egg on top of the avocado.

7. Top with your favorite toppings, such as sliced tomatoes, red onion, or hot sauce.

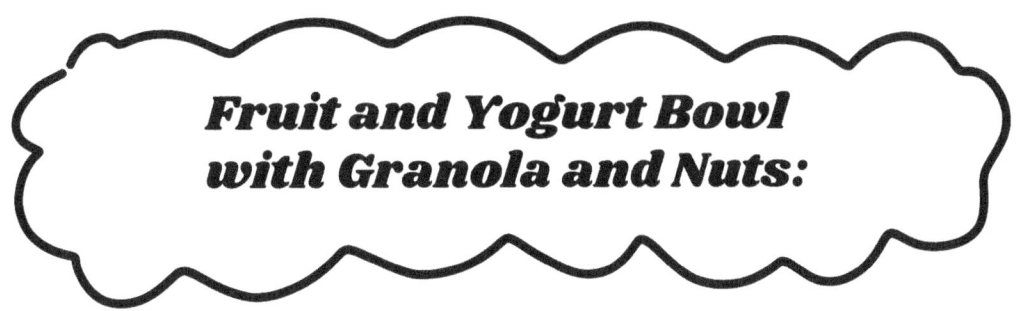

Fruit and Yogurt Bowl with Granola and Nuts:

This colorful and flavorful breakfast bowl is a medley of fresh fruits, creamy yogurt, crunchy granola, and nutrient-rich nuts, providing a balance of fiber, protein, and healthy fats.

Recipe

Preparation Time: 5 minutes	Cooking Time: none	Serving Size: 1

Nutritional Information per Serving

Calories: 300, Protein: 10g, Fat: 10g Carbohydrates: 40g, Fiber: 5g, Sugar: 15g (without honey or maple syrup)

Ingredients;

- 1/2 cup plain yogurt
- 1/2 cup mixed berries
- 1/4 cup granola
- 1 tablespoon chopped nuts
- Honey or maple syrup to taste (optional)

Instructions:

1. In a bowl, combine yogurt, mixed berries, granola, and chopped nuts.
2. Drizzle with honey or maple syrup to taste, if desired.

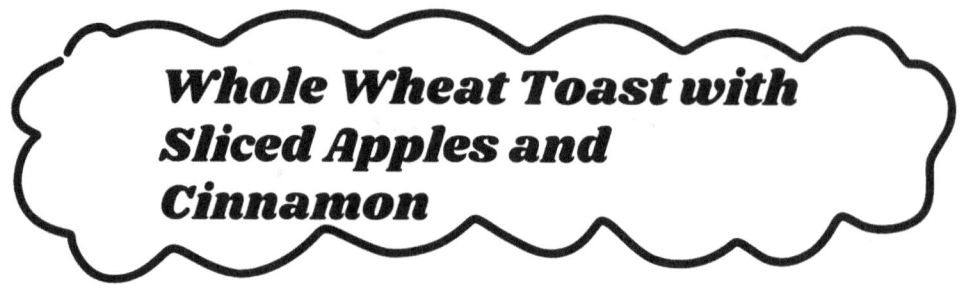

Whole Wheat Toast with Sliced Apples and Cinnamon

This simple yet elegant breakfast combines the sweetness of sliced apples with the warmth of cinnamon, all atop a base of fiber-rich whole wheat toast.

Recipe

Preparation Time: 5 minutes	Cooking Time: 2 minutes	Serving Size: 1

Nutritional Information per Serving

Calories: 200 (without honey or maple syrup), Protein: 6g, Fat: 5g, Carbohydrates: 35g. Fiber: 5g, Sugar: 12g (without honey or maple syrup)

Ingredients;

- 1 slice whole wheat bread
- 1/2 apple, sliced
- 1 teaspoon cinnamon
- Honey or maple syrup to taste (optional)

Instructions:

1. Toast the bread to your desired level of doneness.
2. In a small bowl, combine sliced apples and cinnamon.
3. Spread the apple mixture evenly over the toasted bread.
4. Drizzle with honey or maple syrup to taste, if desired.

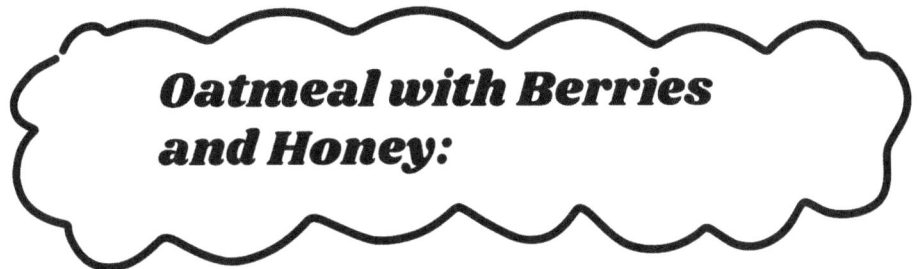

Oatmeal with Berries and Honey:

This comforting and nourishing breakfast option combines the fiber and protein from oats with the antioxidants from berries and the sweetness of honey, providing a sustained energy boost throughout the morning.

Recipe

Preparation Time: 5 minutes	Cooking Time: 5 minutes	Serving Size: 1

Nutritional Information per Serving

Calories: 250, Protein: 5g, Fat: 5g, Carbohydrates: 40g, Fiber: 5g, Sugar: 10g

Ingredients;

- 1/2 cup rolled oats
- 1 cup water or milk
- 1/4 cup mixed berries
- 1 tablespoon honey

Instructions:

1. In a small saucepan, combine oats and water or milk.
2. Bring to a boil over medium heat, then reduce heat and simmer for 5 minutes, or until oats are cooked through.
3. Stir in berries and honey.

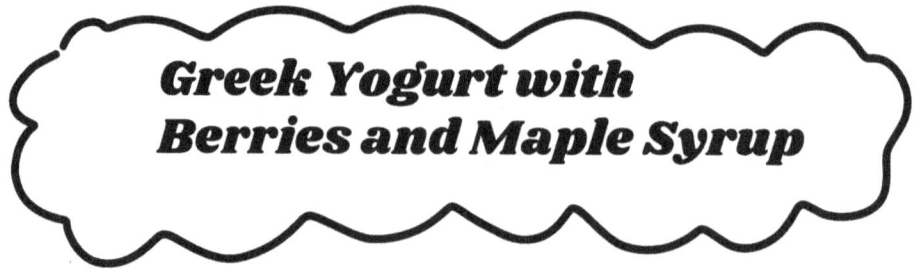

Greek Yogurt with Berries and Maple Syrup

This protein-rich breakfast is a delightful combination of creamy Greek yogurt, vibrant berries, and a touch of sweetness from maple syrup.

Recipe

Preparation Time: 5 minutes	Cooking Time: 5 minutes	Serving Size: 1

Nutritional Information per Serving

Calories: 250, Protein: 15g, Fat: 5g, Carbohydrates: 30g, Fiber: 5g, Sugar: 15g

Ingredients;

- 1 cup plain Greek yogurt
- 1/2 cup mixed berries
- 1 tablespoon maple syrup
- 1 teaspoon vanilla extract

Instructions:

1. In a small bowl, combine Greek yogurt, mixed berries, maple syrup, and vanilla extract.
2. Stir gently to combine.

Lunch

Enjoy satisfying and flavorful DASH-approved lunches

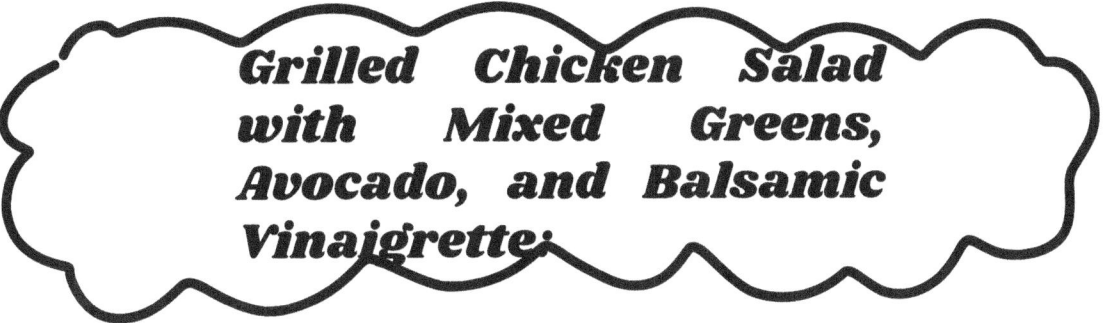

Grilled Chicken Salad with Mixed Greens, Avocado, and Balsamic Vinaigrette;

This salad is a refreshing and nutritious option, combining the protein from grilled chicken with the healthy fats from avocado and the antioxidants from mixed greens, all drizzled with a tangy balsamic vinaigrette.

Recipe

Preparation Time: 15 minutes	Cooking Time: 10 minutes	Serving Size: 12

Nutritional Information per Serving

Calories: 450, Protein: 45g Fat: 25g Carbohydrates: 25g Fiber: 5g Sugar: 15g

Ingredients;
For the Dressing:
- 1/4 cup extra-virgin olive oil
- 3 tablespoons balsamic vinegar
- 2 teaspoons honey
- 1/2 teaspoon salt
- 1/4 teaspoon black pepper

Ingredients
For the Salad;
- 2 boneless, skinless chicken breasts
- 4 cups mixed greens
- 1 avocado, sliced
- 1/2 cup cherry tomatoes, halved
- 1/4 cup crumbled feta cheese
- 1/4 cup chopped walnuts

Instructions

1. Make the dressing: In a small bowl, whisk together the olive oil, balsamic vinegar, honey, salt, and pepper.
2. Marinate the chicken: Place the chicken breasts in a resealable plastic bag or shallow dish. Pour half of the dressing over the chicken, making sure to coat it evenly. Marinate for at least 30 minutes, or up to 4 hours.
3. Grill the chicken: Preheat a grill or grill pan to medium heat. Grill the chicken for 4-5 minutes per side, or until cooked through.
4. Assemble the salad: In a large bowl, combine the mixed greens, avocado, tomatoes, feta cheese, and walnuts.
5. Drizzle the remaining dressing over the salad.
6. Slice the grilled chicken and add it to the salad.
7. Toss to coat and enjoy!

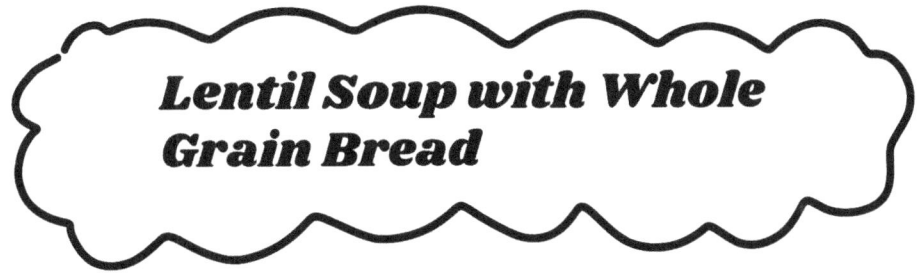

Lentil Soup with Whole Grain Bread

This hearty and satisfying soup is packed with protein and fiber from lentils, while whole grain bread provides additional fiber and complex carbohydrates

Recipe

Preparation Time: 15 minutes	Cooking Time: 30 minutes	Serving Size: 6

Nutritional Information per Serving

Per serving (1 cup soup with 2 slices whole grain bread):
Calories: 450 Protein: 20gFat: 10g Carbohydrates: 70g Fiber: 15g
Sugar: 10g

Ingredients;

For the Soup:

- 1 cup dried green lentils, rinsed
- 1 tablespoon olive oil
- 1 onion, chopped
- 2 carrots, chopped
- 2 celery stalks, chopped
- 2 cloves garlic, minced
- 1 teaspoon cumin
- 1/2 teaspoon paprika
- 1 teaspoon dried oregano
- 6 cups vegetable broth
- 1 (14.5-ounce) can diced tomatoes, undrained
- 1 (15-ounce) can tomato sauceSalt and pepper to taste

For Serving:
- Whole grain bread, sliced

Instructions:

- In a large pot, heat the olive oil over medium heat. Add the onion, carrots, and celery, and cook until softened, about 5 minutes.
- Stir in the garlic, cumin, paprika, and oregano. Cook for 1 minute more, until fragrant.
- Add the lentils, vegetable broth, diced tomatoes, and tomato sauce. Bring to a boil, then reduce heat and simmer for 20-30 minutes, or until lentils are tender.
- Season with salt and pepper to taste.
- Serve hot with a slice of whole grain bread.

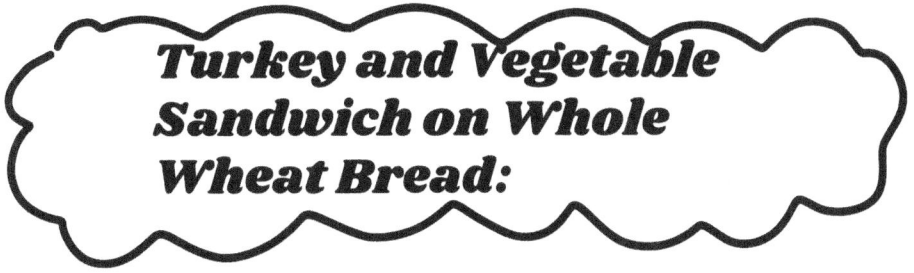

Turkey and Vegetable Sandwich on Whole Wheat Bread:

This classic sandwich is a customizable delight, featuring lean protein from turkey, flavorful vegetables, and the fiber-rich goodness of whole wheat bread.

Recipe

Preparation Time: 5 minutes	Cooking Time: None	Serving Size: 1

Nutritional Information per Serving

Per serving (1 sandwich):   Calories: 540 Protein: 46g Fat: 25g Carbohydrates: 30g Fiber: 4g Sugar: 4g

Ingredients;

- 2 slices whole-wheat bread
- 4 ounces sliced deli turkey breast
- 2 ounces sliced provolone cheese
- 2 green leaf lettuce leaves
- 1 tomato, sliced
- 1/2 cucumber, sliced
- 2 tablespoons mayonnaise

Instructions

1. Spread mayonnaise evenly on one slice of bread.
2. Layer turkey breast, provolone cheese, lettuce, tomato, and cucumber on the other slice of bread
3. Close the sandwich and enjoy!

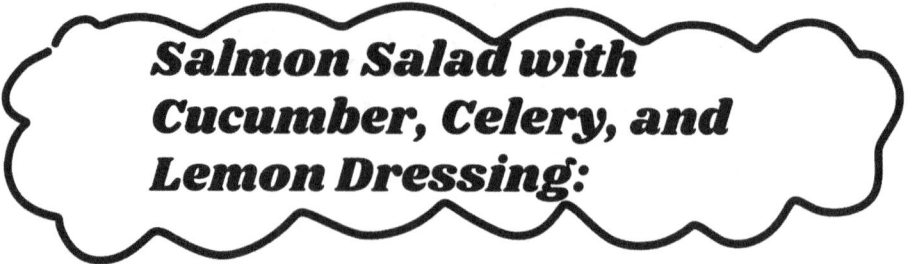

Salmon Salad with Cucumber, Celery, and Lemon Dressing:

This light and flavorful salad combines the omega-3 fatty acids from salmon with the refreshing crunch of cucumber and celery, all enhanced by a zesty lemon dressing.

Recipe

Preparation Time: 10 minutes	Cooking Time: None	Serving Size: 2

Nutritional Information per Serving

Per serving (1 cup salad):   Calories: 250 Protein: 25g Fat: 15g Carbohydrates: 10g Fiber: 2g Sugar: 3g

Ingredients;

For the Salad:

- 4 ounces cooked salmon, flaked
- 1/2 cucumber, diced
- 1/2 celery stalk, diced
- 1/4 cup finely chopped red onion
- 2 tablespoons chopped fresh dillSalt and pepper to taste

Ingredients;

For the Dressing:

- 2 tablespoons lemon juice
- 1 tablespoon olive oil
- 1 teaspoon Dijon mustard
- 1/2 teaspoon dried dillSalt and pepper to taste

Instructions

- In a large bowl, combine the cooked salmon, cucumber, celery, red onion, and dill.
- In a small bowl, whisk together the lemon juice, olive oil, Dijon mustard, dried dill, salt, and pepper.
- Pour the dressing over the salmon mixture and toss to coat.
- Serve immediately on a bed of lettuce or with crackers.

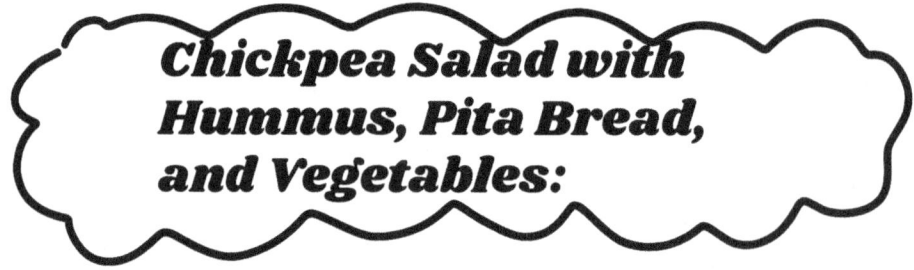

Chickpea Salad with Hummus, Pita Bread, and Vegetables:

This protein-packed and fiber-rich salad features chickpeas, hummus, and a variety of vegetables, served alongside pita bread for a satisfying meal.

Recipe

Preparation Time: 10 minutes	Cooking Time: None	Serving Size: 4

Nutritional Information per Serving

Per serving (1 pita bread with chickpea salad): Calories: 450, Protein: 18g, Fat: 15g.   Carbohydrates: 60g, Fiber: 10g, Sugar: 10g

Ingredients;

For the Chickpea Salad:

- 1 (15-ounce) can chickpeas, rinsed and drained
- 1/4 cup mashed hummus
- 1/4 cup finely chopped red onion
- 1/4 cup chopped cucumber
- 1/4 cup chopped tomato
- 1 tablespoon lemon juice
- 1 tablespoon olive oil
- 1/2 teaspoon dried oregano
- Salt and pepper to taste
- Pita bread, for serving
- Additional vegetables, for serving (optional)

Instructions :

1. In a large bowl, mash the chickpeas with a fork until they are slightly chunky.
2. Add the hummus, red onion, cucumber, tomato, lemon juice, olive oil, oregano, salt, and pepper to the chickpeas and stir until well combined.
3. Toast the pita bread in a toaster or oven until slightly golden brown and warm.
4. Spread the chickpea salad on the pita bread and top with additional vegetables, if desired.
5. Serve immediately and enjoy!

Quinoa Bowl with Black Beans, Corn, and Avocado:

This versatile quinoa bowl is a plant-based powerhouse, offering protein from black beans, fiber from quinoa, and healthy fats from avocado, along with the sweetness of corn.

Recipe

Preparation Time: 10 minutes	Cooking Time: 20 minutes	Serving Size: 2

Nutritional Information per Serving

Per serving: Calories: 350, Protein: 15g, Fat: 10g. Carbohydrates: 50g, Fiber: 8g, Sugar: 5g

Ingredients;

- 1 cup quinoa, rinsed and drained
- 1 (15-ounce) can black beans, rinsed and drained
- 1 (15-ounce) can corn, drained
- 1 ripe avocado, diced
- 1/2 cup chopped red onion
- 1/4 cup chopped cilantro
- 1 tablespoon lime juice
- 1 tablespoon olive oil
- 1/2 teaspoon salt
- 1/4 teaspoon black pepper

Instructions :

1. Cook the quinoa according to package directions.
2. While the quinoa is cooking, combine the black beans, corn, red onion, cilantro, lime juice, olive oil, salt, and pepper in a large bowl.
3. Once the quinoa is cooked, fluff it with a fork and add it to the bowl with the black beans and corn mixture.
4. Stir to combine.
5. Dice the avocado and add it to the bowl.
6. Stir gently.
7. Serve immediately.

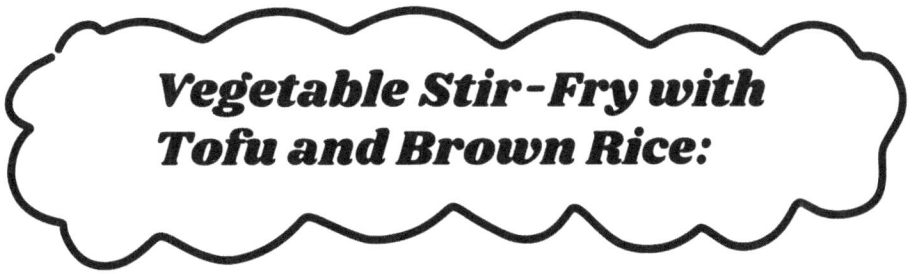

Vegetable Stir-Fry with Tofu and Brown Rice:

This flavorful and nutritious stir-fry is packed with a variety of vegetables, protein from tofu, and complex carbohydrates from brown rice.

Recipe

Preparation Time: 15 minutes	Cooking Time: 20 minutes	Serving Size: 4

Nutritional Information per Serving

Calories: 500, Protein: 30g, Fat: 15g, Carbohydrates: 60g, Fiber: 10g

Ingredients;

- 1 tablespoon olive oil
- 1 onion, chopped
- 2 cloves garlic, minced
- 1 red bell pepper, sliced
- 1 green bell pepper, sliced
- 1 broccoli floret, cut into bite-sized pieces
- 1 cup snow peas
- 1 (14-ounce) block extra-firm tofu, drained and cubed
- 1/4 cup soy sauce
- 1 tablespoon cornstarch
- 3 cups cooked brown rice

Instructions :

1. Heat the olive oil in a large wok or skillet over medium-high heat. Add the onion and cook until softened, about 5 minutes.
2. Add the garlic, red bell pepper, green bell pepper, broccoli, and snow peas. Cook for 5-7 minutes, or until the vegetables are tender-crisp.
3. In a small bowl, whisk together the soy sauce and cornstarch.
4. Add the cubed tofu to the wok or skillet and cook for 5 minutes, or until golden brown.
5. Pour the soy sauce and cornstarch mixture over the tofu and vegetables. Stir to coat.
6. Cook for 2-3 minutes, or until the sauce is thickened.
7. Serve the stir-fry over cooked brown rice.

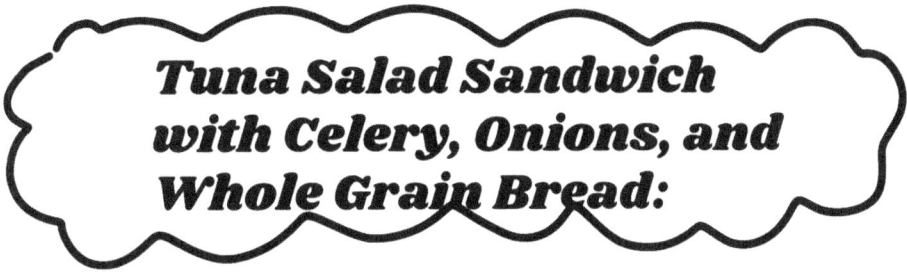

Tuna Salad Sandwich with Celery, Onions, and Whole Grain Bread:

This classic sandwich provides protein from tuna, fiber from celery and onions, and the wholesome goodness of whole grain bread.

Recipe

Preparation Time: 5 minutes	Cooking Time: None	Serving Size: 1

Nutritional Information per Serving

Calories: 400, Protein: 20g, Fat: 15g, Carbohydrates: 45g, Fiber: 5g Sugar: 5g

Ingredients;

- 2 slices whole grain bread
- 3 ounces canned tuna, drained
- 1/4 cup mayonnaise
- 1 tablespoon chopped celery
- 1 tablespoon chopped onion
- Salt and pepper to taste

Instructions :

1. In a medium bowl, flake the tuna with a fork.
2. Add the mayonnaise, celery, onion, salt, and pepper. Stir until combined.
3. Spread the tuna salad evenly on one slice of bread.
4. Top with the other slice of bread.
5. Cut the sandwich in half and enjoy

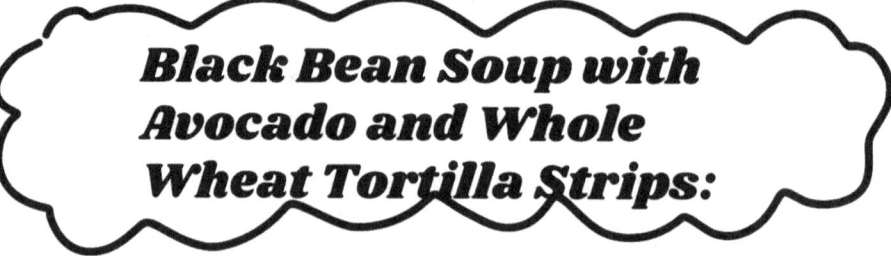

Black Bean Soup with Avocado and Whole Wheat Tortilla Strips:

This hearty and flavorful soup is rich in protein and fiber from black beans, complemented by the creamy texture of avocado and the crunch of whole wheat tortilla strips.

Recipe

Preparation Time: 15 minutes	Cooking Time: 30 minutes	Serving Size: 4

Nutritional Information per Serving

Per serving (1 cup soup with toppings): Calories: 350, Protein: 15g, Fat: 15g   Carbohydrates: 40g, Fiber: 8g, Sugar: 10g

Ingredients;

For the Soup:
- 1 tablespoon olive oil
- 1 onion, chopped
- 2 cloves garlic, minced
- 1 teaspoon ground cumin
- 1/2 teaspoon chili powder
- 1 (15-ounce) can black beans, rinsed and drained
- 1 (14.5-ounce) can diced tomatoes, undrained
- 4 cups vegetable broth
- 1/2 teaspoon salt
- 1/4 teaspoon black pepper

For the Toppings:
- 1 ripe avocado, diced
- 1 cup whole wheat tortilla strips
- 1/4 cup chopped cilantro
- Lime wedges

Instructions;

1. In a large pot, heat the olive oil over medium heat. Add the onion and cook until softened, about 5 minutes.
2. Add the garlic, cumin, and chili powder and cook for 1 minute more, until fragrant.
3. Stir in the black beans, diced tomatoes, vegetable broth, salt, and pepper.
4. Bring to a boil, then reduce heat and simmer for 20-30 minutes, or until the soup has thickened.
5. While the soup is simmering, prepare the toppings. Dice the avocado and cut the tortilla strips into bite-sized pieces. Chop the cilantro.
6. To serve, ladle the soup into bowls. Top with avocado, tortilla strips, cilantro, and a squeeze of lime juice.

Lentil Burgers with Lettuce, Tomato, and Onion on Whole Wheat Buns:

These lentil burgers offer a plant-based alternative to traditional burgers, providing protein and fiber from lentils, while whole wheat buns add extra fiber and complex carbohydrates.

Recipe

Preparation Time: 20 minutes	Cooking Time: 30 minutes	Serving Size: 4

Nutritional Information per Serving

Per serving (1 burger with toppings):   Calories: 450, Protein: 15g, Fat: 15g   Carbohydrates: 60g, Fiber: 10g, Sugar: 10g

Ingredients;

For the Lentil Burgers;
- 1 cup dried green lentils, rinsed
- 1 onion, finely chopped
- 2 cloves garlic, minced
- 1 carrot, finely chopped
- 1 celery stalk, finely chopped
- 1/4 cup chopped fresh parsley
- 1 teaspoon ground cumin
- 1/2 teaspoon smoked paprika
- 1/4 cup rolled oats
- 1 tablespoon olive oil
- Salt and pepper to taste

For the Toppings:
- 4 whole wheat buns
- Lettuce leaves
- Tomato slices
- Onion slices
- Ketchup or mustard (optional)

Instructions;

1. Preheat the oven to 375 degrees F (190 degrees C).
2. In a large pot, bring the lentils to a boil. Reduce heat to low and simmer for 20 minutes, or until the lentils are tender. Drain and set aside.
3. In a large skillet, heat the olive oil over medium heat. Add the onion, garlic, carrot, and celery and cook until softened, about 5 minutes.
4. Stir in the cumin, paprika, and cooked lentils.
5. Mash the lentil mixture with a fork until it is slightly chunky.
6. Stir in the rolled oats, salt, and pepper.
7. Form the lentil mixture into 4 patties.
8. Place the patties on a baking sheet lined with parchment paper.
9. Bake for 20 minutes, or until the patties are cooked through.
10. While the patties are baking, toast the buns.
11. To assemble the burgers, place a lettuce leaf on the bottom bun. Top with a lentil patty, tomato slices, onion slices, and ketchup or mustard, if desired.
12. Top with the bun lid and enjoy!

Chicken Caesar Salad with Grilled Chicken, Romaine Lettuce, Parmesan Cheese, and Caesar Dressing:

This salad is a flavorful twist on a classic, combining the protein from grilled chicken with the crispness of romaine lettuce, the savory notes of Parmesan cheese, and the tangy dressing.

Recipe

Preparation Time: 15 minutes	Cooking Time: 20 minutes	Serving Size: 4

Nutritional Information per Serving

Per serving (1 salad with 4 ounces of grilled chicken): Calories: 450, Protein: 45g, Fat: 20g, Carbohydrates: 25g, Fiber: 5g, Sugar: 10g

Ingredients;

For the Dressing:

- 1/4 cup extra-virgin olive oil
- 3 tablespoons balsamic vinegar
- 2 teaspoons lemon juice
- 1 teaspoon anchovy paste
- 1 clove garlic, minced
- 1/2 teaspoon grated Parmesan cheese
- 1/4 teaspoon salt
- 1/4 teaspoon black pepper

For the Salad:

- 4 boneless, skinless chicken breasts
- 1 head of romaine lettuce, chopped
- 1/2 cup shaved Parmesan cheese
- 1/4 cup croutons

Instructions;

1. Make the dressing: In a small bowl, whisk together the olive oil, balsamic vinegar, lemon juice, anchovy paste, garlic, Parmesan cheese, salt, and pepper.
2. Marinate the chicken: Place the chicken breasts in a resealable plastic bag or shallow dish. Pour half of the dressing over the chicken, making sure to coat it evenly. Marinate for at least 30 minutes, or up to 4 hours.
3. Grill the chicken: Preheat a grill or grill pan to medium heat. Grill the chicken for 4-5 minutes per side, or until cooked through.
4. Assemble the salad: In a large bowl, combine the romaine lettuce, shaved Parmesan cheese, and croutons.
5. Drizzle the remaining dressing over the salad.
6. Slice the grilled chicken and add it to the salad.
7. Toss to coat and enjoy!

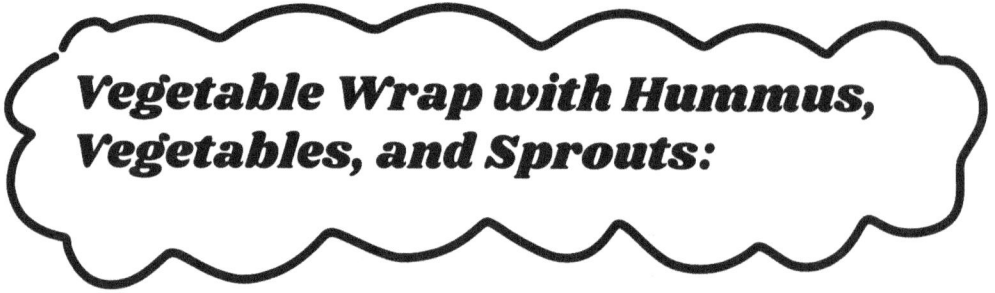

Vegetable Wrap with Hummus, Vegetables, and Sprouts:

This versatile wrap is a convenient and nutritious option, featuring hummus for protein, vegetables for fiber and vitamins, and sprouts for added crunch.

Recipe

Preparation Time: 5 minutes	Cooking Time: none	Serving Size: 1

Nutritional Information per Serving

Calories: 350, Protein: 10g, Fat: 15g Carbohydrates: 40g, Fiber: 10g, Sugar: 10g

Ingredients;

For the Dressing:
- 1 large whole-wheat tortilla
- 1/4 cup hummus
- 1/2 cup shredded carrots
- 1/2 cup sliced cucumber
- 1/4 cup sliced tomato
- 1/4 cup alfalfa sprouts

Instructions:

1. Spread the hummus evenly on the whole-wheat tortilla.
2. Layer the carrots, cucumber, tomato, and sprouts on top of the hummus.
3. Roll the tortilla up tightly.
4. Cut the wrap in half and enjoy!

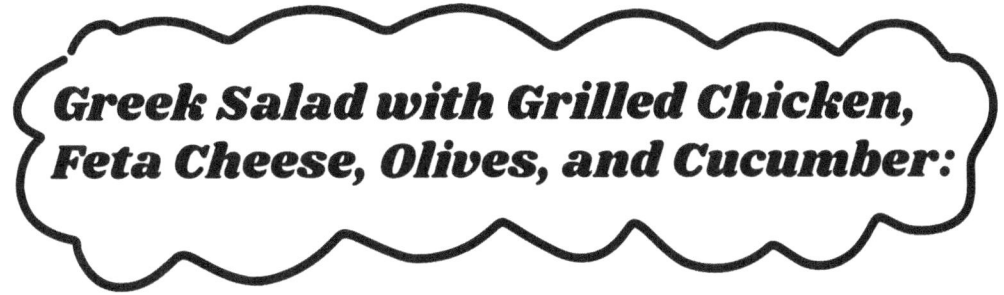

Greek Salad with Grilled Chicken, Feta Cheese, Olives, and Cucumber:

This Mediterranean-inspired salad is a delightful combination of protein from grilled chicken, tangy feta cheese, savory olives, refreshing cucumber, and a light vinaigrette.

Recipe

Preparation Time: 20 minutes	Cooking Time: 10 minutes	Serving Size: 2

Nutritional Information per Serving

Calories: 450, Protein: 45g, Fat: 25g   Carbohydrates: 25g, Fiber: 5g, Sugar: 10g

Ingredients;

For the Salad:
- 1 head of romaine lettuce, chopped (or use a combination of romaine, green leaf, and red leaf lettuce)
- 1 cucumber, thinly sliced
- 1/2 cup cherry tomatoes, halved
- 1/4 cup Kalamata olives, pitted and halved
- 1/4 cup crumbled feta cheese

For the Dressing:
- 1/4 cup olive oil
- 3 tablespoons red wine vinegar
- 1 teaspoon oregano
- 1 clove garlic, minced
- 1/4 teaspoon salt
- 1/4 teaspoon black pepper

For the Chicken:
- 1 boneless, skinless chicken breast
- 1 tablespoon olive oil
- 1 teaspoon oregano
- 1/2 teaspoon salt
- 1/4 teaspoon black pepper

<u>Instructions</u>:
1. Make the dressing: In a small bowl, whisk together the olive oil, red wine vinegar, oregano, garlic, salt, and pepper.
2. Marinate the chicken: In a medium bowl, whisk together the olive oil, oregano, salt, and pepper. Place the chicken breast in the bowl and turn to coat evenly. Marinate for at least 30 minutes, or up to 4 hours.
3. Grill the chicken: Preheat a grill or grill pan to medium heat. Grill the chicken for 4-5 minutes per side, or until cooked through.
4. Assemble the salad: In a large bowl, combine the romaine lettuce, cucumber, cherry tomatoes, Kalamata olives, and feta cheese.
5. Slice the grilled chicken and add it to the salad.
6. Drizzle the dressing over the salad and toss to coat.
7. Serve immediately and enjoy!

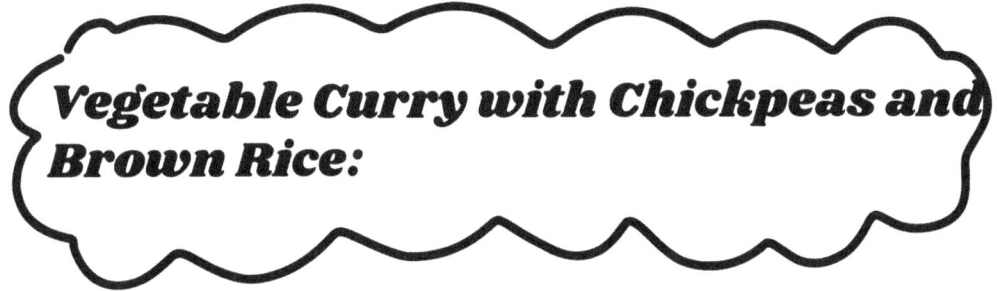

Vegetable Curry with Chickpeas and Brown Rice:

This aromatic curry is a flavorful and nutritious option, featuring chickpeas for protein, a variety of vegetables for fiber and vitamins, and brown rice for complex carbohydrates.

Recipe

Preparation Time: 30 minutes	Cooking Time: 45 minutes	Serving Size: 4

Nutritional Information per Serving

Calories: 500, Protein: 20g, Fat: 15g Carbohydrates: 75g, Fiber: 10g, Sugar: 15g

Ingredients;

For the Curry:
- 1 tablespoon olive oil
- 1 onion, chopped
- 2 cloves garlic, minced
- 1 tablespoon grated ginger
- 1 teaspoon ground cumin
- 1 teaspoon garam masala
- 1/2 teaspoon turmeric
- 1/4 teaspoon chili powder
- 1 (14-ounce) can diced tomatoes, undrained
- 1 (15-ounce) can chickpeas, drained and rinsed
- 1 cup vegetable broth
- Salt and pepper to taste

For the Rice:
- 1 cup brown rice
- 2 cups water

Instructions:

1. Cook the rice: In a medium saucepan, bring the water to a boil. Add the brown rice and reduce heat to low. Simmer for 45 minutes, or until the rice is cooked through.
2. Make the curry: While the rice is cooking, heat the olive oil in a large pot over medium heat. Add the onion and cook until softened, about 5 minutes.
3. Add the garlic, ginger, cumin, garam masala, turmeric, and chili powder and cook for 1 minute more, until fragrant.
4. Stir in the diced tomatoes, chickpeas, and vegetable broth. Bring to a boil, then reduce heat to low and simmer for 20 minutes, or until the flavors have melded.
5. Season the curry with salt and pepper to taste.
6. Serve the curry over the cooked rice.

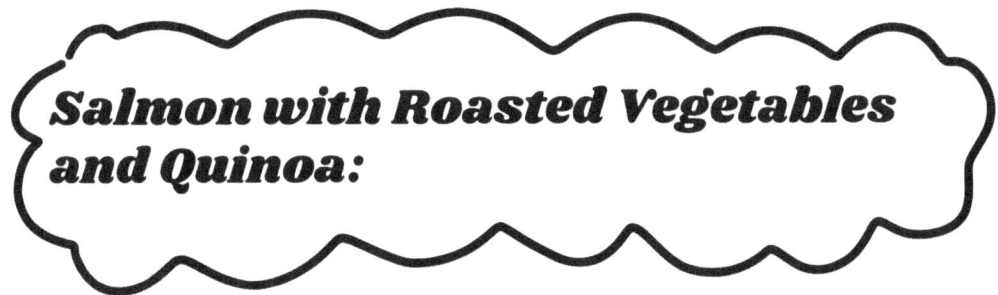

Salmon with Roasted Vegetables and Quinoa:

This balanced meal combines the omega-3 fatty acids from salmon with the nutrient-dense goodness of roasted vegetables and the fiber-rich protein from quinoa.

Recipe

Preparation Time: 20 minutes	Cooking Time: 30 minutes	Serving Size: 2

Nutritional Information per Serving

Per serving (1 salmon filet with roasted vegetables and quinoa):
Calories: 450, Protein: 35g, Fat: 15g, Carbohydrates: 40g, Fiber: 5g, Sugar: 10g

Ingredients;
For the Salmon:
- 2 salmon filets (about 6 ounces each)
- 1 tablespoon olive oil
- 1 teaspoon lemon juice
- 1/2 teaspoon salt
- 1/4 teaspoon black pepper

For the Quinoa:
- 1 cup quinoa, rinsed and drained
- 1 1/2 cups water
- 1/2 teaspoon salt

For the Roasted Vegetables:
- 1 tablespoon olive oil
- 1 red onion, chopped
- 1 green bell pepper, chopped
- 1 yellow squash, diced
- 1 zucchini, diced
- 1/2 teaspoon salt
- 1/4 teaspoon black pepper

Instructions:

1. Preheat the oven to 400 degrees F (200 degrees C).
2. Prepare the salmon: In a small bowl, whisk together the olive oil, lemon juice, salt, and pepper. Drizzle the salmon filets with the marinade and set aside.
3. Prepare the roasted vegetables: In a large bowl, toss together the red onion, green bell pepper, yellow squash, zucchini, salt, and pepper. Drizzle the vegetables with 1 tablespoon of olive oil and toss to coat.
4. Spread the vegetables in a single layer on a baking sheet. Roast for 20 minutes, or until the vegetables are tender and slightly caramelized.
5. Prepare the quinoa: In a medium saucepan, combine the quinoa, water, and salt. Bring to a boil over high heat, then reduce heat to low, cover, and simmer for 15 minutes, or until the quinoa is cooked through and the water is absorbed.
6. While the vegetables and quinoa are cooking, cook the salmon: Heat the remaining 1 tablespoon of olive oil in a large skillet over medium heat. Place the salmon filets skin-side down in the skillet and cook for 5-7 minutes, or until the skin is crispy. Flip the salmon filets and cook for an additional 3-5 minutes, or until cooked to your desired doneness.
7. Fluff the quinoa with a fork.
8. To assemble the dish, divide the quinoa among two plates. Top with the roasted vegetables and salmon filets.
9. Serve immediately and enjoy!

Dinner

Create delectable DASH-inspired dinners for the whole family

Baked Lemon Herb Salmon with Roasted Vegetables:

This vibrant dish combines the omega-3 fatty acids from salmon with the antioxidant-rich goodness of roasted vegetables, all infused with the zesty flavors of lemon and herbs.

Recipe

Preparation Time: 15 minutes	Cooking Time: 25 minutes	Serving Size: 2

Nutritional Information per Serving

Per serving (1 salmon fillet with roasted vegetables): Calories: 400, Protein: 30g, Fat: 15g, Carbohydrates: 30g, Fiber: 5g, Sugar: 5g

Ingredients;

For the Salmon:
- 2 salmon filets (about 6 ounces each)
- 1 tablespoon olive oil
- 1 tablespoon lemon juice
- 1/2 teaspoon dried dill
- 1/2 teaspoon dried oregano
- 1/4 teaspoon salt
- 1/4 teaspoon black pepper

For the Roasted Vegetables:
- 1 tablespoon olive oil
- 1 red onion, chopped
- 1 green bell pepper, sliced
- 1 carrot, chopped
- 1 zucchini, sliced
- 1/2 teaspoon salt
- 1/4 teaspoon black pepper

Instructions:

1. Preheat the oven to 400 degrees F (200 degrees C).
2. Prepare the salmon: In a small bowl, whisk together the olive oil, lemon juice, dill, oregano, salt, and pepper. Drizzle the salmon filets with the marinade and set aside.
3. Prepare the roasted vegetables: In a large bowl, toss together the red onion, green bell pepper, carrot, zucchini, salt, and pepper. Drizzle the vegetables with 1 tablespoon of olive oil and toss to coat.
4. Spread the vegetables in a single layer on a baking sheet. Roast for 15 minutes.
5. Remove the baking sheet from the oven and place the salmon filets on top of the vegetables. Return the baking sheet to the oven and roast for an additional 10 minutes, or until the salmon is cooked through and the vegetables are tender.
6. Serve immediately and enjoy!

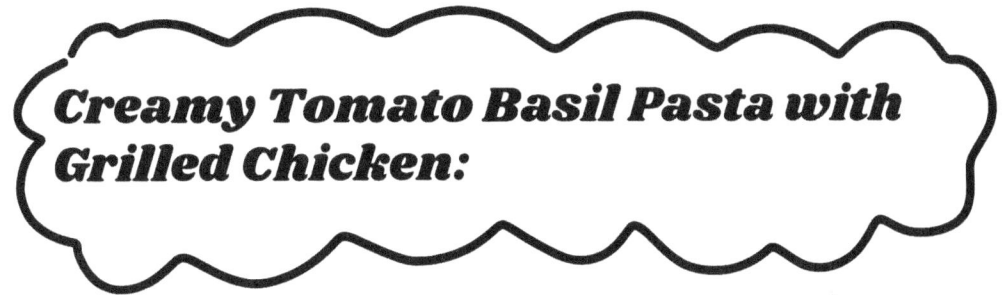

Creamy Tomato Basil Pasta with Grilled Chicken:

This comforting pasta dish features a creamy tomato basil sauce, protein-rich grilled chicken, and whole wheat pasta for a balanced and satisfying meal.

Recipe

Preparation Time:	Cooking Time:	Serving Size:

Nutritional Information per Serving

Calories: 550, Protein: 40g, Fat: 20g, Carbohydrates: 60g, Fiber: 10g, Sugar: 10g

Ingredients;

For the Grilled Chicken:
- 2 boneless, skinless chicken breasts
- 1 tablespoon olive oil
- 1 teaspoon dried oregano
- 1/2 teaspoon salt
- 1/4 teaspoon black pepper

For the Pasta:
- 1 pound pasta (such as penne, farfalle, or fusilli)

For the Creamy Tomato Basil Sauce:
- 2 tablespoons olive oil
- 1 onion, chopped
- 2 cloves garlic, minced
- 1 (14.5-ounce) can diced tomatoes, undrained
- 1/2 cup heavy cream
- 1/4 cup chopped fresh basil
- 1/2 teaspoon salt
- 1/4 teaspoon black pepper

Instructions:

1. Marinate the chicken: In a medium bowl, whisk together the olive oil, oregano, salt, and pepper. Place the chicken breasts in the bowl and turn to coat evenly. Marinate for at least 30 minutes, or up to 4 hours.
2. Grill the chicken: Preheat a grill or grill pan to medium heat. Grill the chicken for 4-5 minutes per side, or until cooked through.
3. Make the creamy tomato basil sauce: While the chicken is grilling, heat the olive oil in a large saucepan over medium heat. Add the onion and cook until softened, about 5 minutes.
4. Add the garlic and cook for 1 minute more, until fragrant.
5. Stir in the diced tomatoes and bring to a simmer.
6. Reduce heat to low and simmer for 10 minutes, or until the sauce has thickened.
7. Stir in the heavy cream, chopped basil, salt, and pepper.
8. Cook the pasta: In a large pot of boiling salted water,
9. cook the pasta according to package directions.
10. Drain the pasta and add it to the sauce. Toss to coat.
11. Slice the grilled chicken and add it to the pasta.
12. Serve immediately and enjoy!

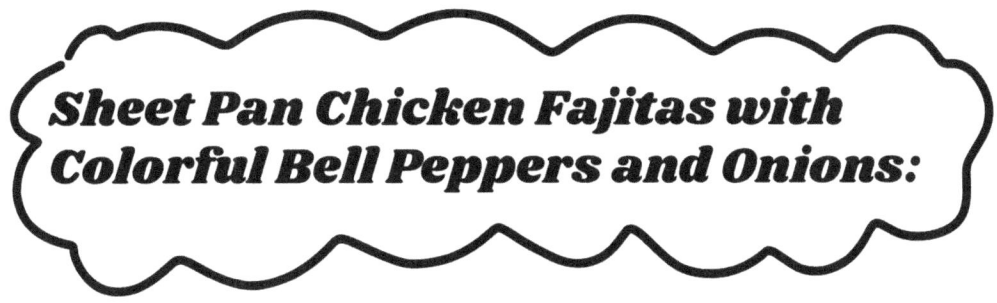

Sheet Pan Chicken Fajitas with Colorful Bell Peppers and Onions:

This sizzling fajita fiesta brings together tender chicken, flavorful bell peppers, and savory onions, all cooked to perfection on a single sheet pan for easy cleanup.

Recipe

Preparation Time: 15 minutes	Cooking Time: 20 minutes	Serving Size: 4

Nutritional Information per Serving

Per serving (2 chicken fajitas with toppings): Calories: 450, Protein: 30g, Fat: 20g, Carbohydrates: 40g, Fiber: 5g, Sugar: 10g

Ingredients;

For the Chicken Fajitas:
- 1 ½ pounds boneless, skinless chicken breasts, sliced into thick strips
- 3 bell peppers (I use green, yellow, and red), cored and sliced into strips
- 1 red onion, thinly sliced
- 2 cloves garlic, minced
- 3 tablespoons olive oil
- 1 lime, juiced
- 1/4 cup fresh cilantro, chopped

For the Toppings:
- 8-10 small flour tortillas
- Sliced avocado or guacamole
- Pico de gallo
- Shredded cheese
- Sour cream

Instructions:

- preheat the oven to 425 degrees F (220 degrees C).
- Place the chicken, peppers, onions, and garlic on a sheet pan. Drizzle with olive oil and lime juice.
- Sprinkle the chicken and vegetables with salt and pepper to taste.
- Toss everything together to coat evenly and spread in a single layer.
- Bake for 15-20 minutes, or until the chicken is cooked through and the vegetables are tender.
- Warm the tortillas in the oven or a skillet.
- To assemble the fajitas, place a chicken fajita on each tortilla.
- Top with avocado or guacamole, pico de gallo, shredded cheese, and sour cream.
- Serve immediately and enjoy!

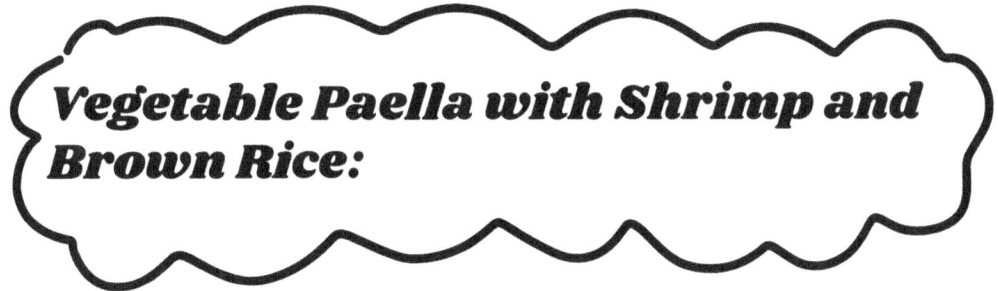

Vegetable Paella with Shrimp and Brown Rice:

This Spanish-inspired paella is a medley of vegetables, protein-packed shrimp, and fiber-rich brown rice, offering a flavorful and nutritious meal.

Recipe

Preparation Time: 25 minutes	Cooking Time: 45 minutes	Serving Size: 4

Nutritional Information per Serving

Calories: 550, Protein: 30g, Fat: 20g, Carbohydrates: 65g, Fiber: 10g, Sugar: 15g

Ingredients;

For the Paella:

- 2 tablespoons olive oil
- 1 onion, chopped
- 2 cloves garlic, minced
- 1 zucchini, chopped
- 1 yellow squash, chopped
- 1 red bell pepper, chopped
- 1 cup chopped tomatoes
- 1 teaspoon smoked paprika
- 1/2 teaspoon turmeric
- 1/4 teaspoon saffron threads
- 2 cups vegetable broth
- 1 cup brown rice
- 1 pound shrimp, peeled and deveined
- 1/2 cup chopped fresh parsley

Instructions:

1. Heat the olive oil in a large paella pan or skillet over medium heat. Add the onion and cook until softened, about 5 minutes.
2. Add the garlic, zucchini, yellow squash, and red bell pepper and cook for 5 minutes more, until the vegetables are tender.
3. Stir in the chopped tomatoes, smoked paprika, turmeric, and saffron threads. Cook for 1 minute more, until fragrant.
4. Pour in the vegetable broth and bring to a boil.
5. Add the brown rice and reduce heat to low. Simmer for 20 minutes, or until the rice is cooked through.
6. Stir in the shrimp and cook for 5 minutes more, until the shrimp are pink and opaque.
7. Sprinkle with chopped parsley and serve immediately.

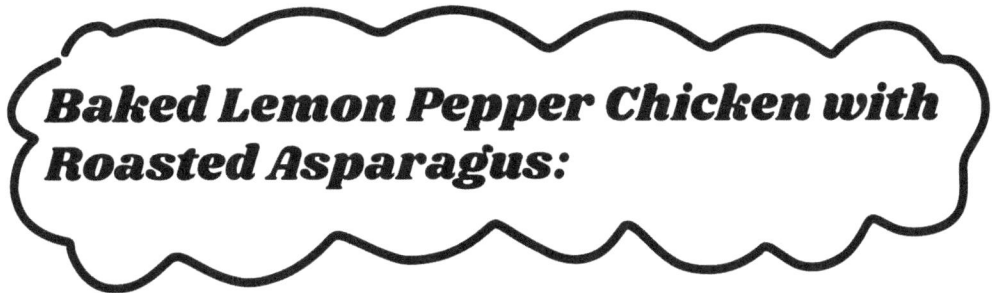

Baked Lemon Pepper Chicken with Roasted Asparagus:

This flavorful and healthy dish features tender chicken seasoned with lemon pepper and roasted asparagus, providing a balance of protein and vegetables.

Recipe

Preparation Time: 15 minutes	Cooking Time: 25 minutes	Serving Size: 4

Nutritional Information per Serving

Per serving (1 chicken breast with asparagus): Calories: 350, Protein: 30g, Fat: 15g, Carbohydrates: 25g, Fiber: 5g, Sugar: 5g

Ingredients;

For the Chicken:
- 4 boneless, skinless chicken breasts (about 6 ounces each)
- 1 tablespoon olive oil
- 2 tablespoons lemon juice
- 1 tablespoon lemon pepper seasoning
- 1/2 teaspoon salt
- 1/4 teaspoon black pepper

For the Asparagus:
- 1 pound asparagus, trimmed
- 1 tablespoon olive oil
- 1/4 teaspoon salt
- 1/4 teaspoon black pepper

Instructions:

1. Preheat the oven to 400 degrees F (200 degrees C).
2. Marinate the chicken: In a small bowl, whisk together the olive oil, lemon juice, lemon pepper seasoning, salt, and pepper. Place the chicken breasts in the bowl and turn to coat evenly. Marinate for at least 30 minutes, or up to 4 hours.
3. Prepare the asparagus: Preheat a large baking sheet with parchment paper.
4. Drizzle the asparagus with olive oil and season with salt and pepper.
5. Spread the asparagus in a single layer on the baking sheet.
6. Bake the chicken and asparagus: Place the baking sheet in the oven and bake for 15 minutes.
7. Remove the baking sheet from the oven and place the chicken breasts on top of the asparagus.
8. Return the baking sheet to the oven and bake for an additional 10 minutes, or until the chicken is cooked through and the asparagus is tender.
9. Serve immediately and enjoy!

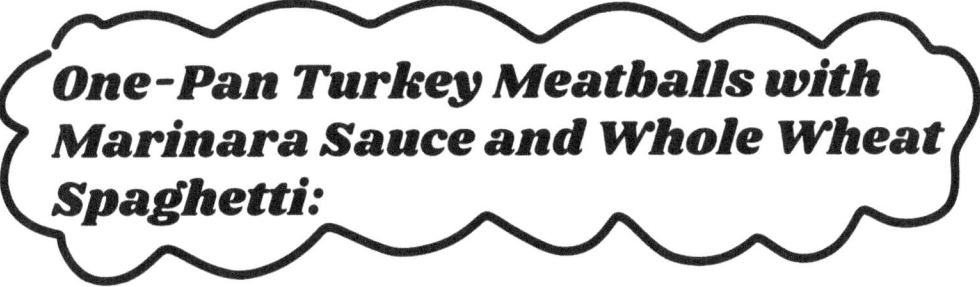

One-Pan Turkey Meatballs with Marinara Sauce and Whole Wheat Spaghetti:

These juicy turkey meatballs are simmered in a flavorful marinara sauce and served over whole wheat spaghetti for a family-friendly favorite.

Recipe

Preparation Time: 20 minutes	Cooking Time: 30 minutes	Serving Size: 4

Nutritional Information per Serving

Per serving (1 serving of meatballs, sauce, and spaghetti):
Calories: 500, Protein: 40g, Fat: 20g, Carbohydrates: 60g, Fiber: 10g, Sugar: 10g

Ingredients;

For the Meatballs:
- 1 pound ground turkey
- 1/2 cup bread crumbs
- 1/4 cup grated Parmesan cheese
- 1 egg
- 1 tablespoon olive oil
- 1/2 teaspoon dried oregano
- 1/4 teaspoon salt
- 1/4 teaspoon black pepper

For the Sauce:
- 1 (14.5-ounce) can diced tomatoes, undrained
- 1 (15-ounce) can tomato sauce
- 1/2 teaspoon dried basil
- 1/4 teaspoon salt
- 1/4 teaspoon black pepper

For the Spaghetti:
- 1 pound whole wheat spaghetti

Instructions:

1. Preheat the oven to 375 degrees F (190 degrees C).
2. Make the meatballs: In a large bowl, combine the ground turkey, breadcrumbs, Parmesan cheese, egg, olive oil, oregano, salt, and pepper. Mix well until combined.
3. Form the meatball mixture into 1-inch balls.
4. Make the sauce: In a large oven-safe baking dish, combine the diced tomatoes, tomato sauce, basil, salt, and pepper.
5. Add the meatballs to the sauce and toss to coat.
6. Cook the meatballs and sauce: Bake for 20 minutes.
7. Cook the spaghetti: While the meatballs and sauce are cooking, cook the spaghetti according to package directions. Drain and set aside.
8. Serve: Once the meatballs and sauce are cooked through, add the cooked spaghetti to the baking dish and toss to coat.
9. Divide the meatballs and spaghetti among four plates and serve immediately.

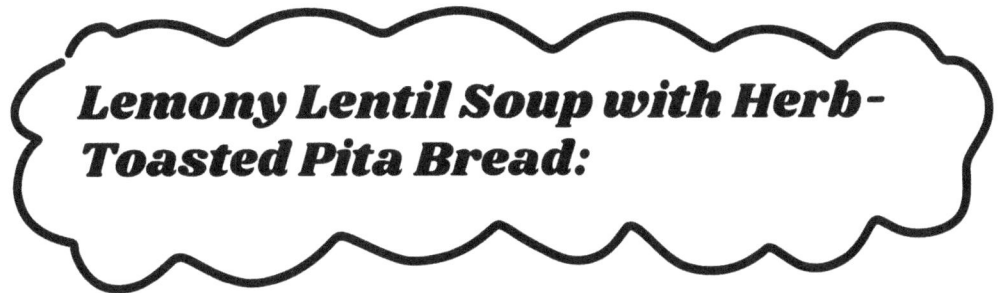

Lemony Lentil Soup with Herb-Toasted Pita Bread:

This hearty and flavorful lentil soup is packed with protein and fiber, while herb-toasted pita bread adds a delightful crunch and extra flavor.

Recipe

Preparation Time: 20 minutes	Cooking Time: 40 minutes	Serving Size: 4

Nutritional Information per Serving

Per serving (1 bowl of soup with 2 slices of herb-toasted pita bread): Calories: 450, Protein: 20g, Fat: 15g, Carbohydrates: 65g, Fiber: 10g, Sugar: 10g

Ingredients;

For the Lentil Soup:
- 2 tablespoons olive oil
- 1 onion, chopped
- 2 cloves garlic, minced
- 1 carrot, diced
- 1 celery stalk, diced
- 1 teaspoon ground cumin
- 1/2 teaspoon smoked paprika
- 1 cup dried green lentils, rinsed
- 4 cups vegetable broth
- 1 (14-ounce) can diced tomatoes, undrained
- 1/4 cup lemon juice
- 1/4 teaspoon salt
- 1/4 teaspoon black pepper
- Fresh parsley, for garnish

For the Herb-Toasted Pita Bread:
- 4 pita breads
- 1/4 cup olive oil
- 1 tablespoon dried oregano
- 1 teaspoon dried basil
- 1/2 teaspoon salt
- 1/4 teaspoon black pepper

Instructions:

1. Make the herb-toasted pita bread: In a small bowl, whisk together the olive oil, oregano, basil, salt, and pepper.
2. Brush the pita bread slices with the herb oil mixture.
3. Place the pita bread slices on a baking sheet and bake at 375 degrees F (190 degrees C) for 5-7 minutes, or until golden brown and crispy.
4. Make the lentil soup: Heat the olive oil in a large pot over medium heat. Add the onion and cook until softened, about 5 minutes.
5. Add the garlic, carrot, and celery and cook for 5 minutes more, until the vegetables are tender.
6. Stir in the cumin and paprika and cook for 1 minute more, until fragrant.
7. Add the lentils, vegetable broth, diced tomatoes, lemon juice, salt, and pepper. Bring to a boil, then reduce heat to low and simmer for 30 minutes, or until the lentils are tender.
8. Serve the lentil soup in bowls garnished with fresh parsley and a side of herb-toasted pita bread.

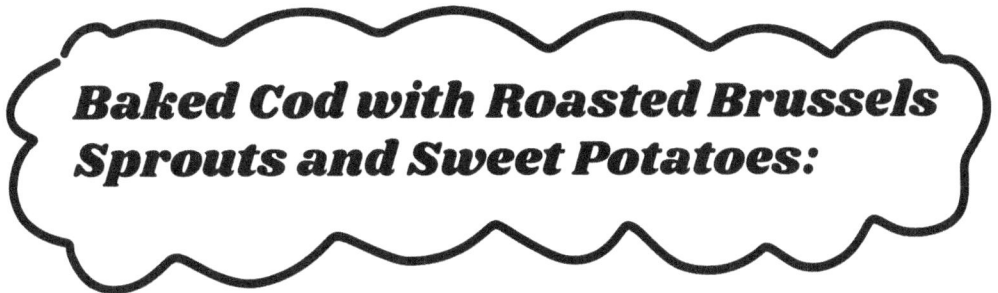

Baked Cod with Roasted Brussels Sprouts and Sweet Potatoes:

This nutritious and flavorful dish combines the protein from cod with the antioxidants from roasted Brussels sprouts and the sweetness of roasted sweet potatoes.

Recipe

Preparation Time: 15 minutes	Cooking Time: 30 minutes	Serving Size: 2

Nutritional Information per Serving

Per serving (1 cod filet with roasted vegetables):   Calories: 450, Protein: 40g, Fat: 20g, Carbohydrates: 40g, Fiber: 5g, Sugar: 10g

Ingredients;

For the Cod:
- 2 cod filets (about 6 ounces each)
- 1 tablespoon olive oil
- 1 tablespoon lemon juice
- 1/2 teaspoon salt
- 1/4 teaspoon black pepper

For the Roasted Vegetables:
- 1 tablespoon olive oil
- 1 pound Brussels sprouts, trimmed and halved
- 1 pound sweet potatoes, peeled and cut into 1-inch chunks
- 1/2 teaspoon salt
- 1/4 teaspoon black pepper

Instructions:

1. Preheat the oven to 400 degrees F (200 degrees C).
2. Marinate the cod: In a small bowl, whisk together the olive oil, lemon juice, salt, and pepper. Place the cod filets in the bowl and turn to coat evenly. Marinate for at least 30 minutes, or up to 4 hours.
3. Prepare the roasted vegetables: In a large bowl, toss together the Brussels sprouts, sweet potatoes, salt, and pepper. Drizzle with 1 tablespoon of olive oil and toss to coat.
4. Spread the vegetables in a single layer on a baking sheet.
5. Bake the cod and vegetables: Place the baking sheet in the oven and bake for 15 minutes.
6. Remove the baking sheet from the oven and place the cod filets on top of the vegetables.
7. Return the baking sheet to the oven and bake for an additional 10 minutes, or until the cod is cooked through and the vegetables are tender.
8. Serve immediately and enjoy!

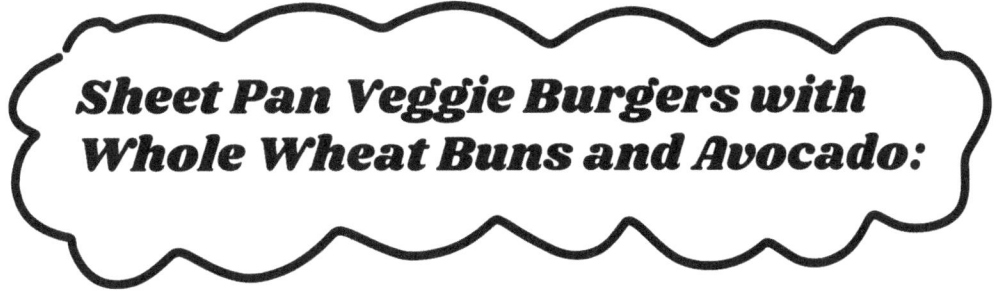

Sheet Pan Veggie Burgers with Whole Wheat Buns and Avocado:

These vegetable burgers are a plant-based alternative to traditional burgers, offering a blend of vegetables, protein from beans, and the healthy fats from avocado.

Recipe

| Preparation Time: 30 minutes | Cooking Time: 20 minutes | Serving Size: 4 |

Nutritional Information per Serving

Per serving (1 veggie burger with whole wheat bun and avocado): Calories: 550, Protein: 30g, Fat: 20g, Carbohydrates: 60g, Fiber: 10g, Sugar: 10g

Ingredients;

For the Veggie Burgers:
- 1 (15-ounce) can chickpeas, drained and rinsed
- 1 (14.5-ounce) can diced tomatoes, undrained
- 1/2 cup chopped red onion
- 1/4 cup chopped fresh parsley
- 1/4 cup chopped fresh cilantro
- 1 tablespoon olive oil
- 1 teaspoon ground cumin
- 1/2 tcaspoon smoked paprika
- 1/4 teaspoon salt
- 1/4 teaspoon black pepper
- 1/2 cup whole wheat bread crumbs

For the Avocado Topping:
- 1 avocado, mashed
- 1/4 cup chopped fresh cilantro
- 1 tablespoon lime juice
- Salt and pepper to taste

For the Whole Wheat Buns:
- 8 slices whole-wheat bread
- 1/4 cup olive oil
- 1 tablespoon dried oregano
- 1 teaspoon dried basil
- 1/2 teaspoon salt
- 1/4 teaspoon black pepper

<u>Instructions</u>:

1. Preheat the oven to 400 degrees F (200 degrees C).
2. Make the veggie burgers: In a large bowl, mash the chickpeas with a fork. Stir in the diced tomatoes, red onion, parsley, cilantro, olive oil, cumin, smoked paprika, salt, and pepper.
3. Add the bread crumbs and mix well until the mixture is firm enough to form patties.
4. Form the veggie burger mixture into 4 equal patties.
5. Make the whole wheat buns: In a small bowl, whisk together the olive oil, oregano, basil, salt, and pepper.
6. Brush the bread slices with the herb oil mixture.
7. Place the bread slices on a baking sheet and bake for 5-7 minutes, or until golden brown and crispy.
8. Assemble the burgers: Place the veggie burgers on a baking sheet and bake for 10 minutes, or until heated through.
9. Make the avocado topping: In a small bowl, mash the avocado with the cilantro, lime juice, salt, and pepper.
10. Serve: To assemble the burgers, place a veggie burger on each toasted bun. Top with a dollop of avocado topping and enjoy!

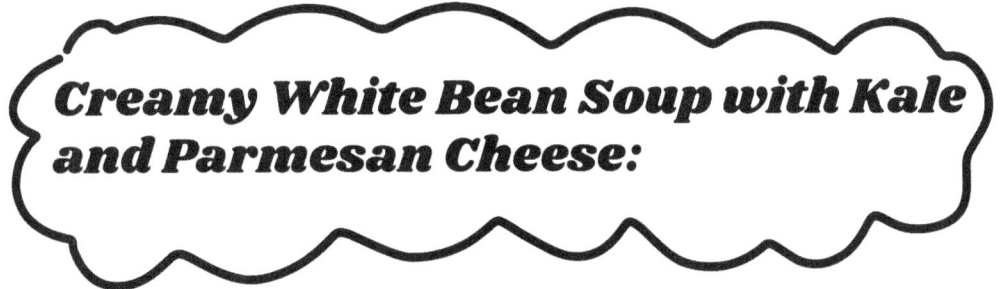

Creamy White Bean Soup with Kale and Parmesan Cheese:

This comforting white bean soup is rich in protein and fiber, while kale adds vitamins and minerals, and Parmesan cheese provides a savory touch.

Recipe

Preparation Time: 15 minutes	Cooking Time: 30 minutes	Serving Size: 4

Nutritional Information per Serving

Per serving (1 cup of soup): Calories: 300, Protein: 15g, Fat:10g Carbohydrates: 40g, Fiber: 10g, Sugar: 10g

Ingredients;

For the Soup:
- 2 tablespoons olive oil
- 1 onion, chopped
- 2 cloves garlic, minced
- 1 carrot, diced
- 1 celery stalk, diced
- 4 cups vegetable broth
- 1 (15-ounce) can cannellini beans, drained and rinsed
- 1 (14.5-ounce) can diced tomatoes, undrained
- 1/2 cup heavy cream
- 1/4 cup chopped fresh kale
- 1/4 cup grated Parmesan cheese
- 1 teaspoon dried oregano
- 1/2 teaspoon salt
- 1/4 teaspoon black pepper

Instructions:

1. Heat the olive oil in a large pot over medium heat. Add the onion and cook until softened, about 5 minutes.
2. Add the garlic, carrot, and celery and cook for 5 minutes more, until the vegetables are tender.
3. Stir in the vegetable broth, cannellini beans, diced tomatoes, heavy cream, kale, Parmesan cheese, oregano, salt, and pepper.
4. Bring to a boil, then reduce heat to low and simmer for 20 minutes, or until the kale is tender.
5. Serve immediately and enjoy!

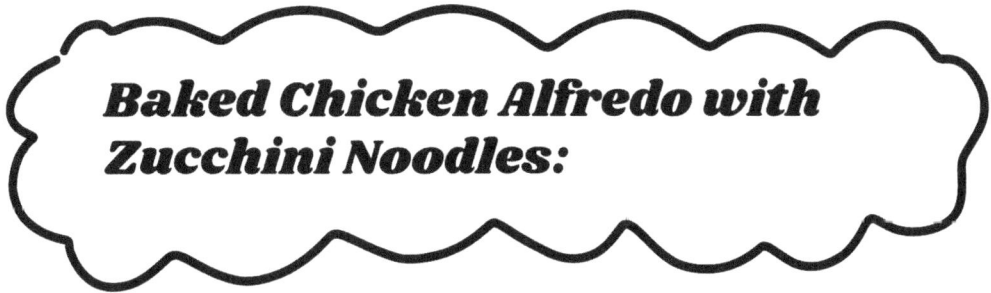

Baked Chicken Alfredo with Zucchini Noodles:

This lightened-up version of chicken Alfredo features zucchini noodles instead of pasta, reducing carbohydrates and adding extra vegetables.

Recipe

Preparation Time: 20 minutes	Cooking Time: 30 minutes	Serving Size: 2

Nutritional Information per Serving

Serving size: 2 chicken breasts Calories: 500, Protein: 45g, Fat: 30g, Carbohydrates: 20g, Fiber: 5g, Sugar: 5g

Ingredients;

Chicken
- 1 lb skinless boneless chicken breasts
- Salt and pepper to taste
- 1 tsp paprika
- ½ tsp garlic powder
- 2 tbsp olive oil

Zucchini noodles
- 1 large zucchini
- 1 tbsp olive oil
- Salt and pepper to taste

Sauce:
- 2 tbsp olive oil
- 1 onion, chopped
- 2 cloves garlic, minced
- ½ tsp dried oregano
- ½ tsp dried basil
- ¼ cup shredded Parmesan cheese
- 1 ½ cups heavy cream

Garnish:
- ¼ cup chopped fresh parsley

Instructions:

Chicken

1. Preheat the oven to 375 degrees F (190 degrees C).
2. Cut the chicken breasts into strips and season with salt, pepper, paprika, and garlic powder.
3. Heat 1 tablespoon of olive oil in a large skillet over medium heat.
4. Add the chicken strips and cook until golden brown and cooked through, about 5-7 minutes per side.
5. Remove the chicken from the skillet and set aside.

Sauce

- In the same skillet, heat the remaining tablespoon of olive oil over medium heat.
- Add the onion and cook until softened, about 5 minutes.
- Add the garlic, oregano, and basil and cook for 1 minute more, until fragrant.
- Stir in the Parmesan cheese and heavy cream.
- Bring to a simmer and cook for 5 minutes, or until the sauce has thickened.

Zucchini noodles

1. Spiralize the zucchini into noodles.
2. Heat 1 tablespoon of olive oil in a large skillet over medium heat.
3. Add the zucchini noodles and cook for 3-5 minutes, or until tender-crisp.
4. Season with salt and pepper to taste.
5. Assemble
6. Add the chicken and zucchini noodles to the sauce and toss to coat.
7. Pour the mixture into a greased baking dish.
8. Bake for 15-20 minutes, or until heated through and bubbly.
9. Garnish with chopped parsley and serve immediately.
10.

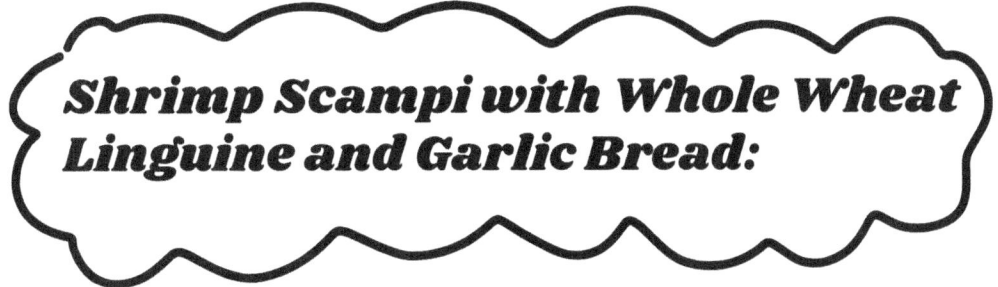

Shrimp Scampi with Whole Wheat Linguine and Garlic Bread:

This classic seafood dish combines tender shrimp with a buttery garlic sauce and whole wheat linguine for a satisfying meal.

Recipe

Preparation Time: 15 minutes	Cooking Time: 20 minutes	Serving Size: 4

Nutritional Information per Serving

Per serving: 500 calories, Protein: 30 grams, Fat: 20 grams, Carbohydrates: 60 grams, Fiber: 10 grams, Sugar: 10 grams

Ingredients;

For the Garlic Bread:
- 1 loaf French bread, sliced
- 2 tablespoons olive oil
- 1 clove garlic, minced
- 1/4 teaspoon dried oregano
- 1/4 cup grated Parmesan cheese

For the Whole Wheat Linguine:
- 12 ounces whole wheat linguine
- Salt to taste
- 1 tablespoon olive oil

For the Shrimp Scampi:
- 1 pound large shrimp, peeled and deveined
- 3 tablespoons olive oil
- 4 cloves garlic, minced
- 1/2 teaspoon dried oregano
- 1/4 teaspoon crushed red pepper flakes
- 1/4 cup dry white wine
- 1/4 cup chopped fresh parsley
- 1/4 cup grated Parmesan cheese
- Salt and pepper to taste

Instructions;

For the Shrimp Scampi:

1. Heat the olive oil in a large skillet over medium heat. Add the garlic and cook for 30 seconds, until fragrant.
2. Add the shrimp and cook for 2-3 minutes per side, until pink and cooked through.
3. Add the oregano, red pepper flakes, wine, parsley, Parmesan cheese, salt, and pepper. Toss to coat.
4. Cook for 1-2 minutes more, until the sauce is thickened.
5. For the Whole Wheat Linguine:
6. Bring a large pot of salted water to a boil.
7. Add the linguine and cook according to package directions.
8. Drain the linguine and toss with 1 tablespoon of olive oil.

For the Garlic Bread:

1. Preheat the oven to 375 degrees F (190 degrees C).
2. In a small bowl, combine the olive oil, garlic, oregano, and Parmesan cheese.
3. Brush the mixture onto the bread slices.
4. Bake for 5-7 minutes, or until golden brown.

To Assemble:

1. Divide the linguine among four plates.
2. Top each plate with shrimp scampi.
3. Serve with garlic bread on the side.

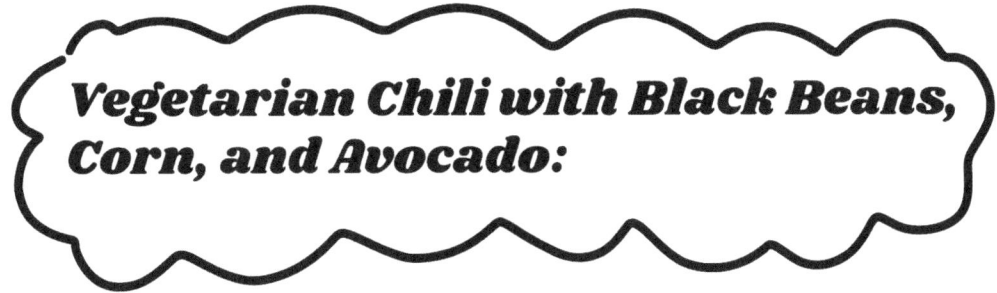

Vegetarian Chili with Black Beans, Corn, and Avocado:

This hearty and flavorful vegetarian chili is packed with protein from black beans, fiber from corn, and the healthy fats from avocado.

Recipe

Preparation Time: 20 minutes	Cooking Time: 30 minutes	Serving Size: 4

Nutritional Information per Serving

Calories: 450 calories, Protein: 30 grams, Fat: 20 grams, Carbohydrates: 40 grams, Fiber: 10 grams, Sugar: 10 grams, Serving

Ingredients;

For the Chili:
- 1 tablespoon olive oil
- 1 large onion, finely chopped
- 2 cloves garlic, minced
- 1 green bell pepper, diced
- 1 (14.5-ounce) can diced tomatoes, undrained
- 1 (15-ounce) can black beans, drained and rinsed
- 1 (15-ounce) can kidney beans, drained and rinsed
- 1 cup frozen corn kernels
- 1 tablespoon chili powder

- 1 teaspoon cumin
- 1/2 teaspoon salt
- 1/4 teaspoon black pepper

For the Avocado Topping:
- 1 ripe avocado, diced
- 1/4 cup chopped fresh cilantro
- 1 tablespoon lime juice
- Salt and pepper to taste

<u>Instructions</u>:

1. Heat the olive oil in a large pot over medium heat. Add the onion and cook until softened, about 5 minutes.
2. Add the garlic and bell pepper and cook for 5 minutes more, until the vegetables are tender.
3. Stir in the diced tomatoes, black beans, kidney beans, corn, chili powder, cumin, salt, and pepper. Bring to a simmer and cook for 20 minutes, or until the chili is thickened.
4. While the chili is cooking, prepare the avocado topping. In a small bowl, combine the diced avocado, chopped cilantro, lime juice, salt, and pepper.
5. To serve, ladle the chili into bowls and top with avocado topping. Enjoy!

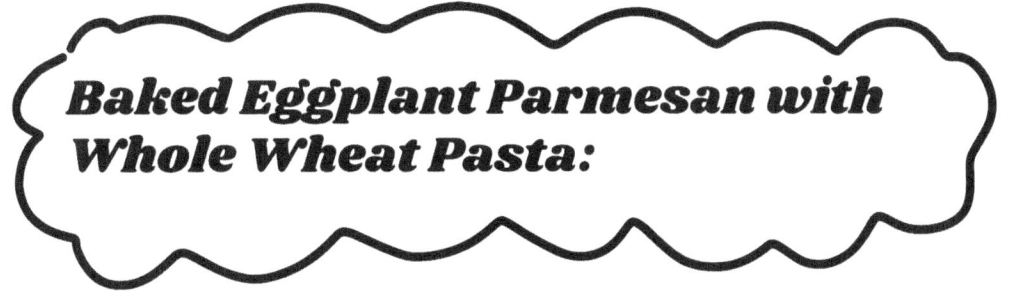

Baked Eggplant Parmesan with Whole Wheat Pasta:

This Italian-inspired dish features eggplant slices breaded and baked with tomato sauce and mozzarella cheese, served alongside whole wheat pasta.

Recipe

Preparation Time: 20 minutes	Cooking Time: 40 minutes	Serving Size: 4

Nutritional Information per Serving

Calories: 500 calories, Protein: 30 grams, Fat: 20 grams, Carbohydrates: 60 grams, Fiber: 10 grams, Sugar: 10 grams

Ingredients;

For the Sauce:
- 2 tablespoons olive oil
- 1 onion, chopped
- 2 cloves garlic, minced
- 1 (14.5-ounce) can diced tomatoes, undrained
- 1 (15-ounce) can tomato sauce
- 1 tablespoon dried oregano
- 1 teaspoon salt
- 1/2 teaspoon black pepper

For the Pasta:
- 1 pound whole wheat pasta
- Salt to taste

For the Eggplant:
- 1 large eggplant, sliced into 1/2-inch rounds
- 1 tablespoon olive oil
- Salt and pepper to taste

For the Topping:
- 1 cup grated Parmesan cheese
- 1/4 cup chopped fresh parsley

Instructions:

1. Preheat the oven to 400 degrees F (200 degrees C).
2. Prepare the eggplant: Spread the eggplant slices in a single layer on a baking sheet. Drizzle with olive oil and season with salt and pepper. Bake for 20 minutes, or until the eggplant is tender.
3. Make the sauce: While the eggplant is baking, heat the olive oil in a large pot over medium heat. Add the onion and cook until softened, about 5 minutes. Add the garlic and cook for 30 seconds more, until fragrant.
4. Stir in the diced tomatoes, tomato sauce, oregano, salt, and pepper. Bring to a simmer and cook for 20 minutes, or until the sauce has thickened.
5. Cook the pasta: Bring a large pot of salted water to a boil. Add the pasta and cook according to package directions.
6. Assemble the dish: Drain the pasta and return it to the pot. Add the sauce and toss to coat.
7. Spread the sauce and pasta mixture in a 9x13-inch baking dish. Top with the eggplant slices and sprinkle with Parmesan cheese.
8. Bake for 20 minutes, or until bubbly and heated through.
9. Garnish with chopped parsley and serve immediately.

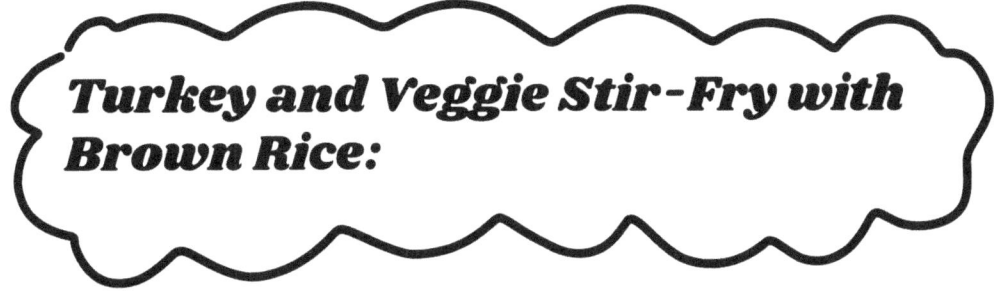

Turkey and Veggie Stir-Fry with Brown Rice:

This flavorful stir-fry combines turkey for protein, a variety of vegetables for fiber and vitamins, and brown rice for complex carbohydrates, making it a well-balanced meal.

Recipe

| Preparation Time: 15 minutes | Cooking Time: 30 minutes | Serving Size: 2 |

Nutritional Information per Serving

Per serving (1 cup brown rice with 1 cup stir-fry): Calories: 400, Protein: 30 grams, Fat: 15 grams, Carbohydrates: 45 grams, Fiber: 5 grams, Sugar: 5 grams

Ingredients;

For the Stir-Fry:
- 1 tablespoon olive oil
- 1 pound ground turkey
- 1 onion, diced
- 2 cloves garlic, minced
- 1 carrot, diced
- 1 celery stalk, diced
- 1 cup broccoli florets
- 1 cup sliced snow peas
- 1/2 cup soy sauce
- 1 tablespoon rice vinegar
- 1 teaspoon sesame oil
- Salt and pepper to taste

For the Brown Rice:
- 1 cup brown rice
- 2 cups water
- Salt to taste

Instructions:

1. Cook the brown rice: In a medium saucepan, combine the brown rice, water, and salt. Bring to a boil, then reduce heat to low and simmer for 45 minutes, or until the rice is cooked through.

2. While the rice is cooking, make the stir-fry: Heat the olive oil in a large skillet or wok over medium-high heat. Add the ground turkey and cook until browned, breaking it up with a spoon.

3. Add the onion, garlic, carrot, and celery and cook for 5 minutes more, until the vegetables are tender.

4. Stir in the broccoli, snow peas, soy sauce, rice vinegar, sesame oil, salt, and pepper. Cook for 5 minutes more, or until the vegetables are crisp-tender.

5. Serve the stir-fry over the cooked brown rice.

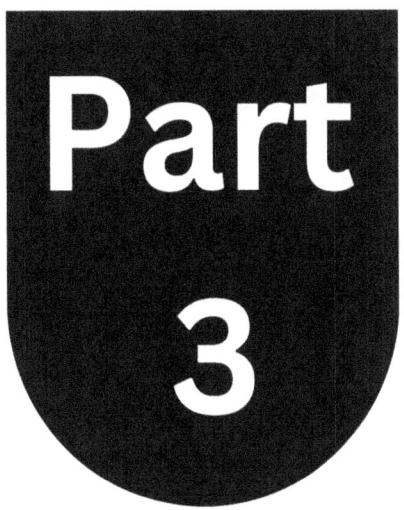

Part 3

Slowing Down the Aging Process with the DASH Diet

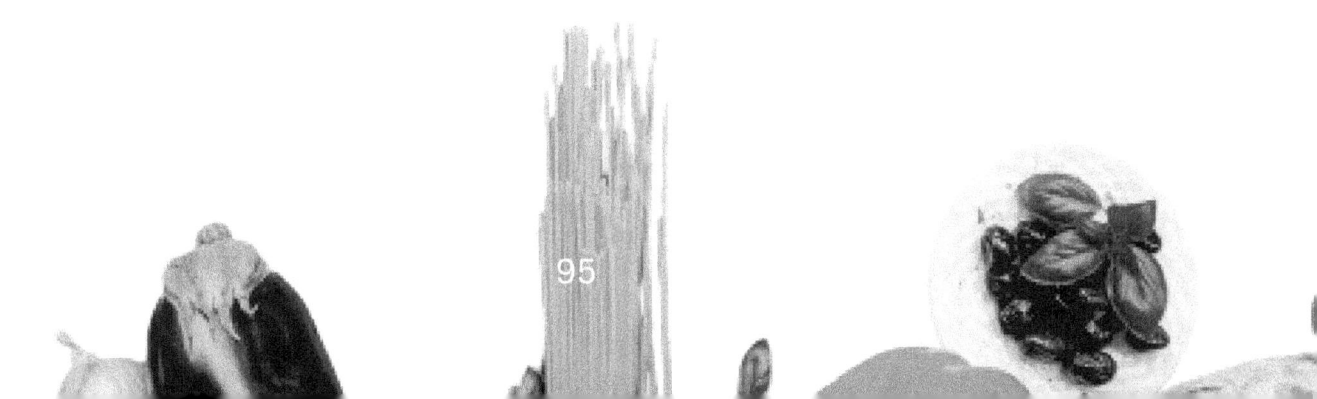

The connection between blood pressure and aging

As we age, our bodies undergo a series of physiological transformations, including the accumulation of cellular damage and the decline of various bodily functions. These changes contribute to an increased risk of age-related diseases, such as cardiovascular disease, stroke, cancer, and dementia.

Among the most significant factors contributing to age-related health problems is high blood pressure. Chronic high blood pressure, also known as hypertension, exerts excessive pressure on the arteries, leading to damage to blood vessels and organs throughout the body. This damage, in turn, increases the risk of cardiovascular diseases, kidney diseases, and cognitive decline.

DASH Diet: A Dietary Approach to Combat Aging and Hypertension

The DASH diet (Dietary Approaches to Stop Hypertension) is a healthy eating plan specifically designed to lower blood pressure. It emphasizes the consumption of fruits, vegetables, whole grains, and low-fat dairy products while limiting saturated and trans fats, sodium, and cholesterol.

The DASH diet's effectiveness in lowering blood pressure stems from its ability to promote favorable changes in various physiological mechanisms, including:

1. **Reduced Sodium Intake**: Sodium, a major component of salt, plays a significant role in regulating blood pressure. By reducing sodium intake, the DASH diet helps to lower blood pressure by promoting fluid balance and reducing fluid retention.

2. **Increased Potassium Intake:** Potassium, a mineral found abundantly in fruits, vegetables, and whole grains, acts as a natural diuretic and counteracts the blood pressure-raising effects of sodium.

3. Enhanced Magnesium Intake: Magnesium, another essential mineral found in DASH-approved foods, helps to relax blood vessels, further contributing to blood pressure reduction.

4. Reduced Saturated and Trans Fats: Saturated and trans fats, commonly found in processed foods and animal products, can contribute to atherosclerosis, the hardening and narrowing of arteries, which in turn increases blood pressure.

5. Increased Fiber Intake: Fiber, abundant in plant-based foods, promotes digestive health and helps to regulate blood sugar levels.

DASH Diet's Impact on Cellular Aging

The DASH diet's benefits extend beyond blood pressure control. It also plays a crucial role in slowing down cellular aging and promoting longevity. Several mechanisms underlie this anti-aging effect:

1. Reduced Oxidative Stress: Oxidative stress, an imbalance between the production of free radicals and the body's ability to neutralize them, contributes to cellular damage and accelerated aging. The DASH diet's abundance of antioxidants, such as vitamins C, E, and beta-carotene, helps to combat oxidative stress and protect cells from damage.

2. Reduced Inflammation: Chronic inflammation, a low-grade immune response, can damage cells and tissues over time. The DASH diet's emphasis on anti-inflammatory foods, such as fruits, vegetables, and whole grains, helps to reduce inflammation and promote healthy aging.

3. Promotes Healthy Gene Expression: The DASH diet has been shown to positively influence the expression of genes involved in cellular repair and longevity.

4. **Reduces DNA Methylation:** DNA methylation, a process that can silence genes, is associated with accelerated aging. The DASH diet's nutrients, such as folic acid and vitamin B12, can help to prevent excessive DNA methylation and promote healthy aging.

Anti-Aging Properties of DASH-Approved Foods

Numerous foods incorporated into the DASH diet are known for their anti-aging properties:

1. **Fruits and Vegetables:** These are packed with antioxidants, vitamins, and minerals that help to protect cells from damage and promote healthy aging.

2. **Whole Grains:** Whole grains are a good source of fiber, which helps to regulate blood sugar levels and reduce inflammation.

3. **Lean Protein:** Lean protein sources, such as fish, poultry, and beans, provide essential amino acids that are needed for cell repair and regeneration.

4. **Low-Fat Dairy:** Low-fat dairy products are a good source of calcium, which is important for bone health and may also help to protect against cognitive decline.

5. **Healthy Fats:** Healthy fats, such as those found in avocados, nuts, and seeds, are beneficial for heart health, brain function, and overall longevity.

Part

4

Boosting Your Immune System with the DASH Diet

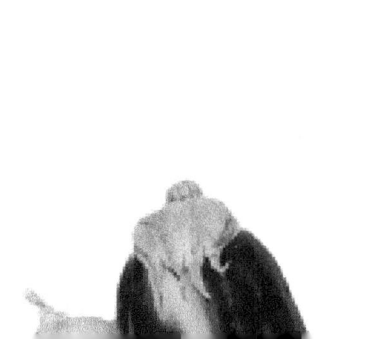
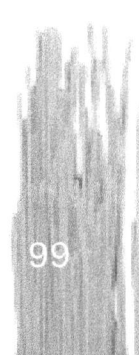
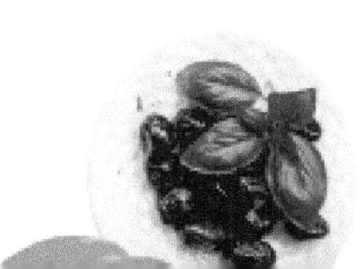

The Role of Nutrition in Immune Function

A well-functioning immune system is essential for maintaining overall health and protecting the body from infections and diseases. Nutrition plays a crucial role in supporting immune function by providing the essential nutrients needed for immune cells to develop, function, and respond effectively to threats.

Essential Nutrients for Immune Health

Several key nutrients are essential for immune system function:

Protein: Protein is the building block of immune cells, providing the amino acids needed to synthesize antibodies, enzymes, and other immune-related molecules.

Vitamin C: Vitamin C is a potent antioxidant that helps protect immune cells from damage caused by free radicals. It also plays a role in collagen synthesis, which is important for maintaining the integrity of the skin and other tissues that act as barriers against pathogens.

Vitamin D: Vitamin D is involved in regulating immune cell activation and function. It also helps to maintain a healthy gut microbiome, which plays a crucial role in overall immune health.

Zinc: Zinc is essential for the development and function of various immune cells, including T cells and B cells. It also plays a role in wound healing and inflammation.

Iron: Iron deficiency can impair immune function by affecting the production of immune cells and their ability to respond to infections.

How the DASH Diet Can Help to Strengthen Your Immune System

The DASH diet, designed to lower blood pressure, also offers benefits for immune system health. By providing a balanced intake of essential nutrients and limiting inflammatory foods, the DASH diet can help to support immune function and reduce the risk of infections.

Anti-Inflammatory Properties of DASH-Approved Foods

Chronic inflammation, often associated with a diet high in processed foods and unhealthy fats, can impair immune function and increase susceptibility to infections. The DASH diet's emphasis on fruits, vegetables, whole grains, and low-fat dairy products helps to reduce inflammation and promote a healthy immune system.

Immune-Boosting Properties of DASH-Approved Foods

Several foods incorporated into the DASH diet are known for their specific immune-boosting properties:

Citrus fruits: Citrus fruits, rich in vitamin C, help protect immune cells from damage and promote antibody production.

Berries: Berries, with their abundance of antioxidants and polyphenols, have been shown to reduce inflammation and enhance immune cell function.

Broccoli: Broccoli contains sulforaphane, a compound that activates enzymes involved in cellular detoxification and protection against infections.

Yogurt: Yogurt, a good source of protein and vitamin D, helps to maintain a healthy gut microbiome and supports immune function.

Nuts and seeds: Nuts and seeds, rich in zinc, vitamin E, and omega-3 fatty acids, contribute to immune cell development and function.

Lifestyle Factors and Immune Health

In addition to diet, several lifestyle factors can influence immune system function:

Regular exercise: Exercise has been shown to boost immune cell activity and reduce the risk of infections.

Adequate sleep: Sleep is crucial for immune system regulation and recovery.

Stress management: Chronic stress can suppress immune function, making it more difficult to fight off infections.

Non-smoking: Smoking can weaken the immune system and increase susceptibility to infections.

Part 5

Putting It All Together: A Practical Guide to Living the DASH Diet

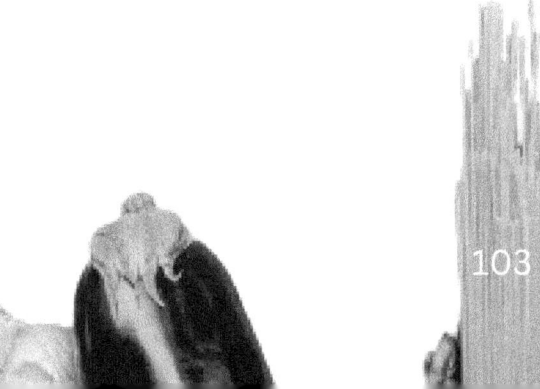

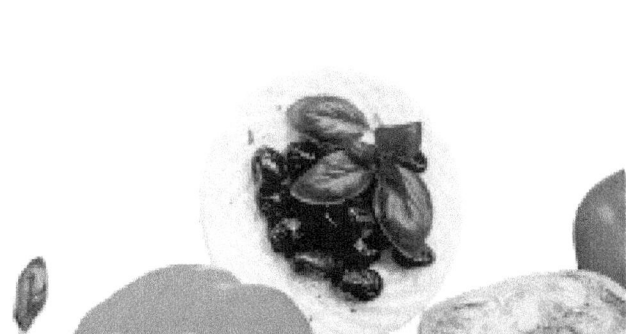

Creating a Personalized DASH Diet Meal Plan

The DASH diet offers flexibility in meal planning, allowing you to tailor it to your individual preferences, dietary needs, and lifestyle. Here's a step-by-step guide to creating your personalized DASH diet meal plan:

1. Assess your current eating habits: Start by evaluating your current food intake to identify areas for improvement. Track your meals and snacks for a few days to gain insights into your food choices, nutrient intake, and potential areas for modification.

2. Set realistic goals: Establish achievable goals for your DASH diet journey. Instead of aiming for drastic changes overnight, focus on making gradual, sustainable improvements.

3. Consider your lifestyle: Adapt your meal plan to fit your daily routine and schedule. If you're often on the go, consider meal prep or incorporating quick and easy DASH-friendly options.

4. Incorporate variety: Choose a variety of foods from each food group to ensure you're getting a balanced intake of nutrients. This will also keep your meals interesting and prevent boredom.

5. Make healthy substitutions: Replace unhealthy ingredients with DASH-friendly alternatives. For instance, switch from full-fat dairy to low-fat or non-fat options, and use whole grains instead of refined grains.

6. Control portion sizes: Practice mindful eating and pay attention to portion sizes. Use smaller plates and bowls to control your intake.

Shopping for DASH-Friendly Ingredients

Equipping your kitchen with DASH-friendly staples will make it easier to plan and prepare nutritious meals. Here are some tips for shopping for

DASH-approved ingredients:

1. Make a list: Plan your meals for the week and create a shopping list to avoid impulse purchases. This will help you stick to your DASH diet goals and prevent overspending.

2. Shop the perimeter of the grocery store: Focus on the outer aisles where fresh produce, whole grains, and lean protein sources are typically found.

3. Choose fruits and vegetables in season: Seasonal produce is often more flavorful and affordable.

4. Read food labels carefully: Pay attention to serving sizes, calorie counts, and sodium content. Choose products with lower sodium content and opt for whole grains over refined grains.

5. Stock up on healthy snacks: Keep DASH-friendly snacks like fruits, vegetables, nuts, and yogurt on hand to avoid unhealthy temptations.

Cooking Techniques for DASH-Approved Meals

Cooking methods can significantly impact the nutritional value and overall healthfulness of your meals. Here are some cooking techniques that align with the DASH diet principles:

1. **Steaming, grilling, baking, and roasting:** These methods use minimal fat and help retain nutrients.

2. **Using herbs and spices for flavor:** Enhance the flavor of your dishes with herbs and spices instead of relying on high-sodium sauces or condiments.

3. **Cooking healthy fats in moderation**: Use healthy fats like olive oil, avocado oil, or nuts in moderation.

4. **Limiting saturated and trans fats**: Avoid processed foods and opt for lean protein sources like fish, poultry, or beans.

5. **Reducing sodium intake:** Use low-sodium ingredients, rinse canned beans, and avoid adding excessive salt to your dishes.

Tips for Maintaining a DASH Diet Lifestyle

Adopting a DASH diet lifestyle involves more than just making changes to your food choices. Here are some tips for maintaining a DASH diet lifestyle:

1. **Make gradual changes:** Instead of overhauling your entire diet overnight, focus on making small, sustainable improvements over time.

2. **Seek support**: Enlist the support of friends, family, or a registered dietitian to help you stay on track and provide encouragement.

3. **Plan ahead**: Plan your meals and snacks for the week to avoid unhealthy choices when hunger strikes.

4. **Cook in bulk**: Prepare larger portions of DASH-friendly meals and freeze them for quick and easy meals later in the week.

5. **Make healthy eating a social activity**: Plan social gatherings around healthy meals and activities.

6. **Reward yourself**: Celebrate your progress and milestones along the way to stay motivated.

7. **Don't be discouraged by setbacks**: Everyone has setbacks. Just get back on track and continue your journey towards a healthier lifestyle.

Conclusion

The DASH diet, with its emphasis on fruits, vegetables, whole grains, and low-fat dairy products, has established itself as a powerful tool for promoting overall health and longevity. By providing a balanced intake of essential nutrients, reducing blood pressure, and strengthening the immune system, the DASH diet empowers individuals to take control of their well-being and embrace a healthier, more vibrant life.

The Power of the DASH Diet for Overall Health and Longevity

The DASH diet's benefits extend far beyond lowering blood pressure. Its positive impact on various aspects of health contributes to a more fulfilling and extended lifespan.

1. Reduced Cardiovascular Disease Risk: By lowering blood pressure, the DASH diet significantly reduces the risk of heart attacks, strokes, and other cardiovascular complications. 80mg

2. Improved Cognitive Function: Studies have shown that the DASH diet can help protect against cognitive decline and reduce the risk of Alzheimer's disease and dementia.

3. Stronger Bones: The DASH diet's emphasis on low-fat dairy products and calcium-rich foods contributes to maintaining bone mineral density and reducing the risk of osteoporosis.

4. Weight Management: The DASH diet's emphasis on nutrient-dense, low-calorie foods can promote healthy weight management and reduce the risk of obesity and its associated health problems.

5. Enhanced Digestive Health: The DASH diet's abundance of fiber promotes digestive health, prevents constipation, and contributes to a healthy gut microbiome.

6. Reduced Inflammation: By reducing inflammation, the DASH diet helps protect against chronic diseases such as arthritis, cancer, and type 2 diabetes.

The Power of the DASH Diet for Overall Health and Longevity

The DASH diet's effectiveness lies in its ability to be integrated into a sustainable lifestyle. By incorporating DASH-friendly foods into your daily routine, adopting healthy cooking techniques, and seeking support from loved ones, you can successfully adopt and maintain this healthy eating pattern.

1. Make Gradual Changes: Instead of drastic overhauls, focus on making small, sustainable changes to your diet and lifestyle over time.

2. Prioritize Meal Planning: Plan your meals for the week to avoid unhealthy choices when hunger strikes. Cook in bulk and freeze portions for quick meals.

3. Incorporate DASH-Friendly Staples: Stock your kitchen with DASH-approved ingredients like fruits, vegetables, whole grains, and lean protein sources.

4. Explore New Recipes: Discover new and exciting DASH-friendly recipes to keep your meals interesting and flavorful.

5. Seek Support: Enlist the help of friends, family, or a registered dietitian to provide encouragement and accountability.

6. Make Healthy Eating a Social Activity: Plan social gatherings around healthy meals and activities, fostering a supportive environment.

7. Reward Yourself: Celebrate your progress and milestones to stay motivated and maintain your commitment to the DASH diet lifestyle.